Small Animal Nutrition

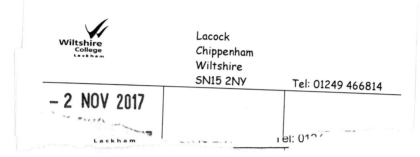

Senior Commissioning Editor: Mary Seager
Desk Editor: Deena Burgess
Development Editor: Caroline Savage
Production Controller: Anthony Read
Cover Designer: Helen Brockway

Small Animal Nutrition

Sandie Agar

Cartoons by Sarah Hough

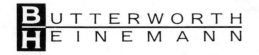

OXFORD AUCKLAND BOSTON JOHANNESBURG MELBOURNE NEW DELHI

First published 2001
 Reprinted 2003, 2004, 2005

ISBN 0 7506 4575 X

British Library Cataloguing in Publication Data
A catalogue record for this book is available from the British Library

Library of Congress Cataloging in Publication Data
A catalog record for this book is available from the Library of Congress

Notice
Medical knowledge is constantly changing. Standard safety precautions
must be followed, but as new research and clinical experience broaden our
knowledge, changes in treatment and drug therapy may become necessary
or appropriate. Readers are advised to check the most current product
information provided by the manufacturer of each drug to be administered
to verify the recommended dose, the method and duration of administration,
and contraindications. It is the responsibility of the practitioner, relying on
experience and knowledge of the patient, to determine dosages and the
best treatment for each individual patient. Neither the Publisher nor the
editors/contributor assumes any liability for any injury and/or damage to
persons or property arising from this publication.

The Publisher

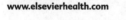
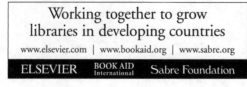
Composition by Genesis Typesetting, Rochester, Kent
Printed and bound in Great Britain by MPG Books Ltd,
Bodmin, Cornwall

Contents

1. Components of food 1

2. Energy 17

7. Clinical nutrition 68

8. Small furries 132

Glossary

abiotic (component): the chemical and physical (non-living) features of an ecosystem.

absorption: the uptake of an ingested substance from the gastrointestinal tract into the villi lining the tract.

acceptability: a measure of whether enough of a food will be eaten to meet the animal's energy requirements.

acidosis: a metabolic imbalance arising from the accumulation of acids or depletion of alkalis from the blood and tissues, resulting in a decreased pH. These animals are described as **acidotic.**

ad lib: ad libitum, unrestricted or freely available.

additive: a substance added to a food for a specific purpose, e.g. colour, flavour, prevention of oxidation.

adipose: fatty.

aerobic: requiring air or free oxygen to live and grow.

alopecia: lack of hair.

amino: the radical –NH2.

anaerobic: able to live and grow without air or free oxygen.

anorexia: the lack or loss of appetite.

anticoagulant: prevents the coagulation of blood.

antioxidant: a substance that prevents the formation of free radicals.

antivitamin: a factor in the diet that degrades or inhibits a vitamin.

arboreal: living in trees.

ascites: the abnormal accumulation of serous fluid in the abdominal cavity.

availability: the amount of a nutrient in food that can be absorbed and utilized by the animal; the difference between the amount ingested and the amount recoverable in the faeces.

BEE: basal energy expenditure.

BER: basal energy requirement.

bile duct: the duct carrying bile from the gall bladder to the duodenum.

biotic (component): the living organisms in an ecosystem.

BMR: basic metabolic rate. The amount of energy required to keep vital organs functioning continuously.

bolus: a rounded mass of food.

borborygmus: pl. borborygmi, rumbling noise produced by movement of gas through the bowel.

brachycephalic: having a short wide head.

buccal or oral cavity: the beginning of the digestive system, includes the mouth and the area between teeth and cheeks.

cachexia: a profound state of general ill health and starvation.

caecotroph or caecotrope: a specialized faecal pellet produced by rabbits and some rodents. Ingestion of these caecotrophs is termed **caecotrophy**.

caecum: the proximal part of the large intestine; its relative size varies between species.

calculolytic food: a food designed to reduce the levels of urolith-forming minerals in the urine.

calculus: mineralized plaque on the surface of a tooth.

Calorie: 1000 calories. One **calorie** (small 'c') is the amount of heat required to raise one gram of water through one degree Celsius

calorimeter: an instrument used to measure the energy content (in the form of heat) of a substance. A fixed amount of the substance is burnt and the heat given off is measured.

carboxyl: the radical –COOH found in organic compounds.

catalyst: a substance which increases the speed of a chemical reaction.

chyle: an emulsion of lymph and triglycerides absorbed into the lacteals during digestion.

chylomicron: a droplet of triglyceride fat together with small amounts of phospholipids and protein absorbed into the lacteals.

chyme: semi-fluid, homogeneous material produced by the mix of gastric juice and ingested food.

cirrhosis: liver disease with loss of normal microscopic lobular structure, replaced by fibrous tissue.

colitis: inflammation of the colon.

colon: that section of the large intestine extending from the caecum to the rectum. It has three sections, the naming of which derives from medical literature. The **ascending colon** begins at the caecum and passes cranially to the right-hand side of the abdominal cavity, crosses to the left-hand side as the **transverse colon** and then passes caudally as the **descending colon**; as it does so it curves in towards the midline and joins the rectum at the **colorectal junction**.

colonocytes: cells lining the colon.

colostrum: the 'first milk' produced for several days before and after parturition; contains maternal antibodies and helps establish passive immunity in the neonates.

conjugated protein: a protein united with a non-protein molecule.

constipation: hard, dry faeces passed infrequently and with difficulty.

crepuscular: appearing or active at dawn and dusk.

cystine: a naturally occurring amino acid sometimes found in the kidneys and urine as hexagonal crystals; forms cystine calculi in the bladder.

cystitis: inflammation of the urinary bladder.

DE: digestible energy; gross energy minus faecal energy.

demineralization: excessive removal of minerals from bone tissues.

DER: daily energy requirement.

dicoumarol: a potent anticoagulant, produced naturally in mouldy clover hay.

digestion: the process of converting food in the gastrointestinal tract into chemical substances which can be absorbed by the body.

diuresis: increased excretion of urine.

dolichocephalic: having a long narrow head.

duodenum: the proximal part of the small intestine, extending from the pylorus to the jejunum. The bile and pancreatic ducts empty into it.

eclampsia: a condition including convulsions and coma.

eicosanoid: a compound derived from arachidonic acid, e.g. prostaglandin.

electrolyte: a chemical substance which, on dissolving in water, separates into electrically charged ions. Many electrolytes are involved in metabolic activities and are essential to the correct functioning of all cells. An **electrolyte imbalance** occurs when the serum concentration of an electrolyte is either too high or too low.

encephalopathy: any degenerative disease of the brain.

energy: the power driving all functions of the living creature. It assumes several forms: chemical, electrical, kinetic, mechanical, radiant or thermal.

energy density: the concentration of energy in a particular food or nutrient.

enteral: referring to the upper alimentary tract.

enteritis: inflammation of the small intestine.

enterocyte: tall columnar cells of the intestinal mucosa, responsible for the absorption of nutrients, electrolytes and water.

enteropathy: any disease of the intestines.

enterotoxin: a toxin specifically affecting the cells of the intestine.

enzyme: a protein acting as a catalyst.

EPI: exocrine pancreatic insufficiency. An inability of the exocrine pancreas to secrete adequate amounts of digestive enzymes.

ester: a compound formed when alcohol is combined with an acid and water is removed.

fermentation: the digestion of nutrients by anaerobic microorganisms.

flatulence: excessive production of gas in the stomach and intestines.

fructo-oligosaccharide: an oligosaccharide containing fructose (fruit sugar) which cannot be hydrolysed by mammalian enzymes and is fermented by some bacteria in the colon.

gall bladder: a reservoir for bile, lying between the lobes of the liver.

gastric reflux: return of the gastric contents to the oesophagus.

GE: gross energy, the total energy content of a food.

glucogenic: producing sugar.

gluconeogenesis: the synthesis of glucose from non-carbohydrate sources.

glucosamine: an amino derivative of glucose found in many glycoproteins and mucopolysaccharides.

gluten: a cereal protein, highest levels in wheat but present in all cereals except rice.

glycerol: a type of alcohol which when linked with fatty acids forms mono-, di- or triglycerides.

glycogen: a polysaccharide, the chief carbohydrate storage material in animals, used as a source of glucose when required. Also called **animal starch**.

glycogenesis: the conversion of glucose to glycogen for storage in the liver.

glycogenolysis: the splitting of glycogen in the liver or muscles to provide glucose.

glycolysis: the enzymatic conversion of glucose to lactate or pyruvate releasing energy, adj. **glycolytic**.

glycosaminoglycans: complex polysaccharides associated with proteins forming an integral part of interstitial fluid, cartilage, skin and tendons, e.g. **chondroitin sulphate**.

haemoglobin: the protein in erythrocytes responsible for transporting oxygen.

heat increment: the heat produced from metabolism of food.

homeostasis: the maintenance of chemical levels and physiological states within narrow margins. Stability which has to be re-established when disease or injury occurs for the animal to regain health.

hormone: a compound acting as a chemical messenger, produced chiefly in the endocrine glands, discharged into capillaries or lymph and transported by the bloodstream to its target organs.

hydrolysis: the splitting of a compound by the addition of water.

hyper-: prefix meaning above, an increase or excessive.

hyperadrenocorticism: disease caused by overactivity of the adrenal cortices.

hypercalcaemia: an excess of calcium in the blood.

hypercalciuria: an excess of calcium in the urine.

hyperglycaemia: an excess of glucose in the blood.

hyperkalaemia: abnormally high levels of potassium in the blood.

hypermetabolism: increased metabolism

hyperparathyroidism: abnormally increased activity of the parathyroid gland.

hyperphosphataemia: excess of phosphates in the blood.

hyperplasia: abnormal increase in the volume of a tissue or organ due to formation of new *normal cells*.

hypertension: persistently high blood pressure.

hypertrophy: increase in volume of a tissue or organ by enlargement of existing cells.

hypo-: prefix meaning below, a decrease or deficient. (Hypo- = low.)

hypoadrenocorticism: reduced hormone production by the adrenal cortex (Addison's disease).

hypocalcaemia: reduced levels of calcium in the blood.

hypocalciuria: reduced levels of calcium in the urine.

hypoglycaemia: abnormally low levels of glucose in the blood.

hypokalaemia: abnormally low levels of potassium in the blood.

hypometabolism: decreased metabolism.

hypophosphataemia: lower than normal levels of phosphates in the blood.

hypothalamus: part of the brain regulating many functions, including endocrine activity, thirst and hunger.

IBD: inflammatory bowel disease.

icterus: jaundice; the yellowing of mucous membranes or skin.

ileocaecal junction: the point at which the ileum and caecum join. The sphincter guarding this junction is the ileocaecal sphincter.

ileum: the distal portion of the small intestine, running from the jejunum to the caecum.

immunocompetence: the ability to develop an immune response after exposure to an antigen.

ingesta: substances taken into the body through the mouth.

integument: skin and hair.

intercostal: between two ribs.

ion: an atom or group of atoms which have an electrical charge. **Cations** are positively charged ions (e.g. sodium Na^+ and potassium K^+). **Anions** are negatively charged ions (e.g. chloride Cl^-).

jejunum: the part of the small intestine extending from the duodenum to the ileum.

joule: the work done by a force of one newton acting over a distance of one metre.

keratinization: the conversion of an active cell into a dead keratinized cell.

ketoacidosis: the accumulation of ketone bodies in the blood resulting in metabolic acidosis.

ketogenic: forming ketone bodies.

ketone: a metabolic product derived from the breakdown of fatty acids. When produced in excess they are excreted in urine. Accumulation in blood and tissues leads to metabolic acidosis. Affected animals are said to be **ketotic**.

lacteal: a capillary of the lymphatic system found within the villus of the small intestine.

lactulose: a disaccharide of galactose and fructose joined by a beta bond. It cannot be hydrolysed by mammalian enzymes but can be fermented by bacteria in the colon.

lignin: a complex structural component of plants usually classed with the carbohydrates, found in wood and straw. It is highly resistant to both enzymatic and chemical degradation.

lipid: a complex organic compound, e.g. fats and oils.

lipoprotein: a large molecular structure comprised of both lipid and protein, responsible for transport of lipids in the blood.

lumen: a cavity or channel within a tubular organ.

lymphangiectasia: dilation of the lymphatic vessels.

matrix: 1. The intercellular substance of a tissue. 2. The organic part of uroliths which remains after the crystalline portion has been dissolved.

MCT: medium-chain trigylceride.

ME: metabolizable energy; the usable energy; digestible energy minus urinary energy.

megaoesophagus: lack of muscle tone and dilation of the oesophagus.

MER: maintenance energy requirements; resting energy requirement plus energy for exercise, digestion and absorption of food.

metabolism: the combination of physical and chemical processes by which living tissue is built up and maintained, **anabolism,** or broken down into smaller components to provide energy, **catabolism**.

metabolite: a substance produced during metabolism.

micelle: an aid to the absorption of fats. A sphere formed from bile salts joined with lipids to create a stable, structured fat droplet in water; they are usually small particles. Emulsion droplets formed by churning actions of the stomach and gut motility are larger.

motility: the ability to move.

mucilage: a gum-like substance in aqueous solution.

multifactorial: arising through the actions of many factors.

myasthenia gravis: muscle weakness, made worse by activity and improved with rest.

myoglobin: the pigment in muscle that transports oxygen.

naris: pl. nares, opening of the nasal cavity.

NE: net energy; metabolizable energy minus the heat increment.

neoplasm: any new and abnormal growth.

nephron: the structural and functional unit of the kidney.

nephrotoxin: a toxin that has a specific effect on the nephrons.

nutrition: the study of the ingestion, assimilation and utilization of food.

obligate: has to be.

obstipation: the passage of soft, watery faeces round a faecal impaction.

OCD: osteochondritis dissecans. Inflammation of bone and cartilage resulting in a piece of articular cartilage splitting or completely separating and falling into the joint space.

oedema: an abnormal accumulation of fluid in the cavities and intercellular spaces of the body.

oesophagitis: inflammation of the oesophagus.

oesophagus: the passage extending from the pharynx to the stomach.

organic compound: a chemical substance containing carbon.

ossification: the formation of bone.

osteodystrophy: any disease of bone where there is failure of the bone to develop normally or abnormal metabolism within mature bone.

osteomalacia: bone softening.

oxidation: a chemical reaction which results in the loss of electrons and leads to an increase of positive charges on an atom or the loss of negative charges. The opposite of this is **reduction** when, as a result of a chemical reaction, electrons are gained. Compounds may, under differing sets of circumstances, act either as electron donors (be oxidized) or as electron acceptors (be reduced). Oxygen is the terminal electron acceptor in mammalian metabolism thus linking food intake and oxygen requirement.

palatability: a measure of how much an animal likes a food.

pancreas: lies in the loop of the duodenum; produces both exocrine and endocrine secretions. The exocrine digestive enzymes are produced by the **acini** (the smallest lobules of a compound gland) and released into the duodenum through the **pancreatic duct(s).** The endocrine hormones are produced in the **islets of Langerhans** (clusters of cells interspersed among the acini).

parenchyma: the functional elements of an organ.

parenteral: not through the alimentary canal.

PEG: percutaneous endoscopic gastrostomy. The placing of a feeding tube from the stomach to the outside of the body wall using an endoscope.

peptide bond: the link which joins two amino acids together. The carboxyl group of one amino acid is linked to the amino group of the next.

peristalsis: a combination of longitudinal and circular muscle movements, producing a wave of contraction which propels the contents of the gastrointestinal tract (or any other tubular structure) on through the system. **Reverse peristalsis** is propulsion in the direction from which the contents have come.

permeable: allowing passage of a material.

pharyngostomy: making an artificial opening into the pharynx.

pharynx: the throat, bifunctional, included in both the respiratory and digestive systems.

pheromones: hormone-like substances secreted by an individual and affecting the behaviour of other members of the same species.

phospholipid: a lipid containing phosphorus, forming the major lipid in cell membranes.

phytin: the calcium and magnesium salt of phytic acid.

pica: depraved appetite.

pododermatitis: inflammation of the skin of the foot.

polydipsia: excessive thirst.

polypeptide: a compound containing two or more amino acids linked by a peptide bond.

polyuria: the formation and excretion of increased volumes of urine.

portosystemic shunt: an abnormality where blood bypasses the liver and passes directly from the portal vein to the systemic circulation.

postprandial: after a meal.

precipitation: the deposition of solid particles from a solution.

precursor: that which 'goes before'. A substance from which another substance may be formed.

protease: any proteolytic enzyme.

proteinaemia: an excess of protein in the blood.

protein-sparing effect: to provide calories predominantly from carbohydrates and fats, thus reducing the need to use protein for energy.

pruritic: itchy.

purine: a constituent of nucleic acid.

radical: a group of atoms. **Free radicals** are extremely reactive radicals which contain an unpaired electron.

rectum: the distal portion of the large intestine lying within the pelvis, extending from the colorectal junction to the anal canal.

regurgitation: the bringing back of undigested food.

RER: resting energy requirement. The energy required by a relaxed animal in a thermoneutral environment, 12 hours after eating.

resorption: reabsorption.

ruga: pl. rugae, a fold or ridge.

saccharide: a carbohydrate, divided into mono-, di-, tri-, oligo- or polysaccharides depending on the number of saccharide groups present.

satiety: having fulfilled all desire to eat and drink.

SCFAs: short-chain fatty acids.

sclera: pl. sclerae, outer coat of the eyeball.

SIBO: small intestinal bacterial overgrowth.

stasis: a ceasing or decrease in flow.

steatorrhoea: excessively fatty faeces.

stomach: curved muscular sac-like enlargement of the alimentary canal between the oesophagus and the duodenum, divided into three parts: proximally the **cardia**, **fundus** or body and **pylorus** distally.

struvite: magnesium-ammonium-phosphate hexahydrate.

substrate: a substance acted on by an enzyme.

supplement: an addition to the basic food.

synthesis: the creation of a compound by the unification of its separate elements.

tenesmus: straining to pass faeces or urine.

tetany: steady contraction of a muscle without twitching

thermoregulation: a physiological process which balances heat production and heat loss in order to maintain body temperature.

TLI: trypsin-like immunoreactivity.

transit time: time taken for food to pass through the digestive tract.

triglyceride: the usual form for fat storage in mammals; an ester of glycerol and three fatty acids.

uraemia: an excess of urea, creatinine and other nitrogenous waste products in the blood; also called **azotaemia**.

urea: the main nitrogenous end product of protein metabolism, formed in the liver from amino acids and ammonia compounds.

urethritis: inflammation of the urethra.

urolith: a calculus in the urine or urinary tract.

urolithiasis: the formation of calculi in the urinary tract.

villus: pl. villi, a small protrusion from the surface of a membrane. **Intestinal villi:** threadlike projections from the mucous membranes lining the small intestine. These provide the sites of absorption for fluids and nutrients.

visceral: relating to the internal organs.

vitamin: a complex organic substance required in small quantities to maintain growth, health and survival of living creatures. Ingestion of excessive amounts leads to **hypervitaminosis**.

Introduction

Food, glorious food

Most of us love food. Food, warmth and shelter are mankind's basic needs. We eat to survive, but food is much more than sustenance, it is an integral part of our lives; a fact that we must not overlook when offering dietary advice.

Food defines nations – paella, pasta, tacos, sushi – and regions within countries. It helps define rank, wealth and culture.

The offering and sharing of food, together with abstinence from it, plays a significant role in virtually all religions. It marks our rites of passage through life – baptisms, marriages and funerals – and frequently plays an important role in the traditions of individual families. It is indelibly linked with memory; mention congealed gravy or lumpy custard and a large proportion of the older generations will instantly recall, with alarming clarity, the school dinners of their youth. In each individual some foods will be linked with feeling secure, being loved and these items will be sought at times of need for the very feelings they invoke. Conversely, foods linked with unhappy memories may be avoided whenever possible.

Eating with friends is more than a sharing of food; dressing up and dining out is a treat, a luxury; feeding a baby, child or pet is an act of love, a giving of far more than sustenance. It is important to the giver that the recipient accepts and enjoys this gift of food.

Food is fun and important, one of life's greatest pleasures; but nutrition, the science of food's inter-action with the body, is regarded as boring by many. However, nutrition can be a fascinating subject. Understanding nutrition involves understanding how any living creature takes the jigsaw that is food caught or offered to it, breaks it up and rebuilds the individual components into a new jigsaw that is the living creature. (In human terms, sausage, mash and baked beans into blood, bone and tissue.) On the way bits are discarded, pieces swopped round and others brought out of storage to complete the picture. It means understanding the fact that, although an animal will eat many times its own weight of food in its lifetime, once it has reached adult body weight that animal will, under most circumstances, maintain that weight, within narrow limits, throughout its life, with only small change in body size and composition.

Nutrition is also a powerful tool in the promotion of good health and longevity as well as the prevention, management and cure of disease. It is a tool that veterinary nurses can use to promote the health and well-being of the animals with which they come into contact. A tool moreover that vets are happy for them to use. Explaining and discussing the role of diet is often time-consuming and time is something that vets are perennially short of. Clients often have queries on diet and a well-informed answer will earn their respect and raise their perception of the value of the nurse and his/her practice. Advice on nutrition is of particular significance when applied to exotics and small furries. Increasing numbers of these animals are being kept as pets and more and more are being seen by vets when problems arise. A large proportion of these problems are directly related to diet and husbandry, and veterinary nurses can do much to help and advise clients on these matters.

I hope the following will prove to you that nutrition, although a complex subject, is not daunting and that at least a few of you who are presently unconvinced will become enthusiastic advisers on diets. But first a little revision.

> Nutrition is a powerful tool in the promotion of good health and prevention of disease.

> Advice on nutrition is of particular significance when applied to exotics and small furries.

The digestive system

In simple organisms such as the amoeba, digestion takes place within a cell – intracellular digestion. In more complex animals, digestion is extracellular – it takes place within the digestive or alimentary tract, outside the cells of the body.

It is important to remember that, although the digestive tract is situated within the animal's body, it is in fact external to that body. This is a difficult concept to grasp, unless one thinks of it as a long convoluted tunnel through the body. The walls of the digestive tract are designed to prevent leakage of gut contents into the body while allowing the passage of nutrients essential to ensure survival of that body. Breakdown in these defences will lead to illness, infection and, if not treated, death.

A factory production line takes individual components and builds them into a finished product, be it a fridge, cooker, car or whatever. The digestive tract is a production line in reverse. It ingests the finished product, moves it along from one breakdown process to the next and finally eliminates the undigested remnants from the body. Food items (and everything else) entering the digestive tract are subject to compression, ripping and shredding, strong acids and alkalis, and enzyme and bacterial attack during this breakdown process, leaving relatively little untouched. Even so some items are more resistant than others and will yield fewer nutrients to the animal than those items which are more easily broken down; of the breakdown products, some are more useful than others. Just to complicate things a little more, different animals have different requirements, some being designed to cope with diets low in nutrients, others having very specific needs. Fortunately, as veterinary nurses we need only concern ourselves with the needs of a small number of animals.

Journey through darkest dog – a tour through the digestive tract

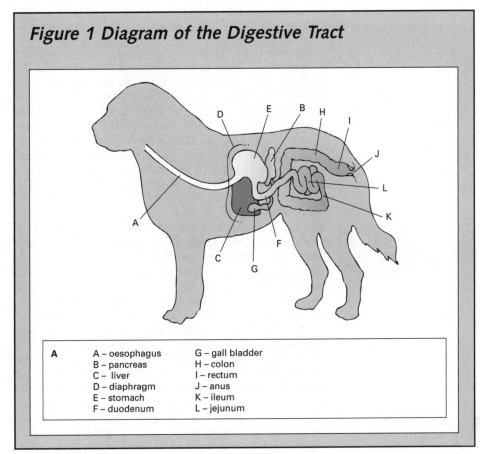

Figure 1 Diagram of the Digestive Tract

A	A – oesophagus	G – gall bladder
	B – pancreas	H – colon
	C – liver	I – rectum
	D – diaphragm	J – anus
	E – stomach	K – ileum
	F – duodenum	L – jejunum

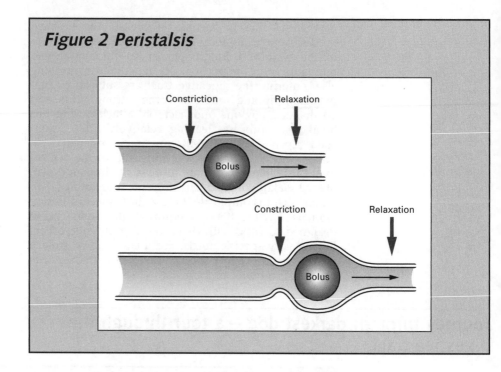

Figure 2 Peristalsis

Food enters the digestive tract through the mouth and is subject to tearing and shredding by the action of the incisors, premolars and molars. The tongue mixes the food with saliva, a mix of water and mucus, which lubricates and softens it, and forms the mix into clumps (boluses) which are propelled into the pharynx and swallowed. The bolus is moved down the chute that is the oesophagus, pushed along by muscles contracting behind it and relaxing ahead of it in a steady peristaltic wave (Figure 2). The way ahead is blocked by a ring of muscle, the cardiac sphincter, but this relaxes as pressure builds up and the bolus is propelled through into a large chamber whose sides are obscured by large folds or rugae. This is the stomach, a muscular bag which acts as a storage organ and food mixer, a sort of biological liquidizer. As the stomach continues to fill and the walls expand, the rugae start to disappear and quantities of liquid flow in from the gastric pits in the stomach walls. This fluid contains hydrochloric acid and enzymes which commence digestion. Churning movements gradually grind the food to a slurry which, mixed with the secretions, becomes chyme. At the lower end of the stomach lies the pyloric sphincter which relaxes at intervals allowing first liquid and then chyme to pass in small quantities through into the first part of the small intestine, the duodenum. Segregation of the diet starts here, with carbohydrate and protein being

The stomach is a biological liquidizer.

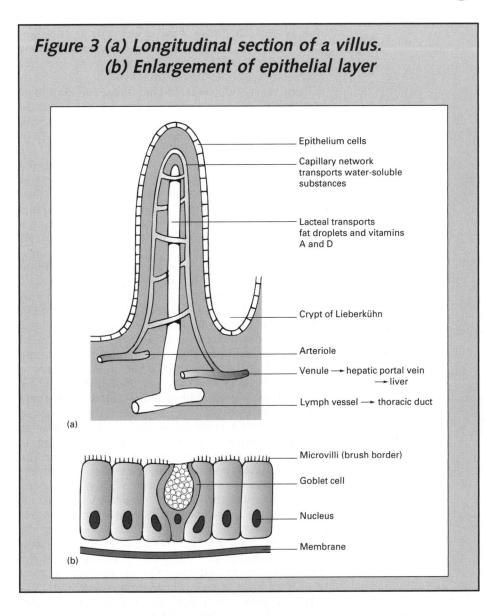

Figure 3 (a) Longitudinal section of a villus. (b) Enlargement of epithelial layer

released first, followed by fat and finally the indigestible material – the content of the food affects the rate of gastric emptying. Colourless fluid enters the duodenum from two ducts coming from the pancreas which lies in the loop made by the first bend of the small intestine. This fluid is alkaline and quickly changes the acidic nature of the chyme to a much more alkaline state. The pancreatic juices also contain powerful enzymes which, in combination with other enzymes produced by glands in the walls of the small intestine, break down the food particles into their smallest components, amino acids, simple sugars, fatty acids and glycerol. Digestion of fats is aided by a yellowish-green fluid, bile, which enters the duodenum from the liver via the bile duct. This emulsifies the fat globules which break up into tiny droplets of oil.

Tides of chyme and fluid pass along the loops and bends of the jejunum and ileum (the second and third parts of the small intestine and lined all the way with finger-like projections – the villi), rather like shoals of small fish swimming through waving fronds of kelp forest on the sea bed (Figure 3). Throughout the passage, the food particles are getting smaller and smaller and then start to diminish in number as they are absorbed through the walls of the villi into the capillaries and lacteals that lie in each one. Every ten seconds or so the villi contract, becoming shorter and fatter, followed by relaxation to their normal shape. This movement aids the passage of absorbed food into the blood and lymphatic systems.

At the end of the ileum, most of what remains consists of indigestible material, dead cells from the intestinal walls, some vitamins and minerals and water. Here another muscular ring, the ileocaecal sphincter, controls the passage of material to the large intestine and the remnants of the food pass into a much larger, smoother passage, the colon, avoiding the small cul-de-sac which is the caecum. (In some other animals as we shall see later, the caecum is expanded into a large organ playing a vital role in digestion.) Ingesta travelling through the colon is propelled first upwards then across the body in the ascending transverse colon. In these sections propulsion becomes a two-way system with reverse peristalsis at intervals directing the ingesta back the way it came. During this time, water and electrolytes are absorbed through the walls of the colon and the residue becomes drier and more compacted. Finally, powerful movements sweep the remains down the descending colon towards the rectum where they await expulsion at an appropriate moment.

With a system so complicated it is easy to see why things go wrong. Perhaps it is more surprising that things function so well most of the time. It is easy to see as well, that many of the functions are influenced by the content of the food eaten. This is the basic idea behind clinical nutrition and will be looked at in detail later, but first we need to understand more about the individual components of food and the uses to which the body puts them.

Components of food

INTRODUCTION

As we have seen, the digestible parts of the ingested food are broken down to their smallest units. These are then able to pass through the wall of the gastrointestinal tract into the body of the animal where they will be used in the multiplicity of functions that sustain life. The indigestible portions of the food remain in the gut where they are either utilized by the bacteria that colonize the various sections or pass through relatively unchanged.

Food comes in many forms, from muscle meat to plant leaf, but all food is composed of some or all of six basic components – water, protein, fat, carbohydrate, vitamins and minerals. These components are often divided into two groups, energy producing (protein, fat and carbohydrate) and non-energy producing (water, vitamins and minerals).

All six have an essential part to play within the animal's body, some being required in large amounts, some only in minute quantities, but excess or deficiency, if maintained over a period of time, will often lead to nutritional disorders and problems for the animal.

Each individual, depending on species, gender, age, physical state and environment, has its own requirements for the different components in varying proportions and it is the nutritionist's challenge to provide a balanced diet to suit the individual animal. To do this we need to know more of each nutrient – its sources and its importance to the animal.

Food:

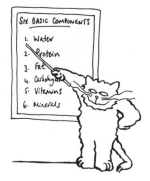

SIX BASIC COMPONENTS
1. Water
2. Protein
3. Fat
4. Carbohydrate
5. Vitamins
6. Minerals

The primary requirement for mammals and other animals is oxygen.

WATER

The primary requirement for mammals and other animals is oxygen; without it they quickly die. Their next requirement is for water, which is regarded as the most important nutrient.

> The most important nutrient is water.

The mammalian body consists of around 70% water and relatively small losses can cause problems. (The proportion of water in newborns is between 75 and 80% and in mature animals between 50 and 60% because of a natural increase in body fat.) An animal may lose almost all its fat and half of its protein but still survive; a loss of 10% water will cause serious illness and a 15% loss will lead to death if not quickly replaced.

Sources

- Ingested water – fluids drunk or eaten in food.
- Metabolic water – produced in the body by oxidation of protein, fat and carbohydrate. This normally supplies around 10% of the daily water requirement and is particularly important to birds and desert animals.

Required for

Water is found throughout the body, both within (intracellular) and without the cells (extracellular) and it is involved in almost all the processes which take place in the body. It is:

- the medium in which the chemical reactions of metabolism take place, e.g. the synthesis of new cell materials and the detoxification of wastes
- a chemical reactant, e.g. hydrolysis of other nutrients
- a lubricant for body tissues
- a transport medium carrying soluble materials and waste products
- the circulatory medium for blood and lymph cells
- involved in temperature control – panting (the principal method of thermoregulation in dogs) causes the evaporation of water from the tongue.

The daily water requirement in healthy animals in millilitres is approximately equal to its daily energy requirements in kilocalories.

> The daily water requirement in healthy animals in millilitres is approximately equal to its daily energy requirements in kilocalories.

PROTEIN

Proteins are organic compounds made from one or more polypeptide chains consisting of amino acids linked together by peptide bonds. There are 23 naturally occurring amino acids and, as these may be joined in any sequence, there is an almost infinite variety of proteins possible. Proteins can also combine with non-protein substances to form conjugated proteins, e.g. haemoglobin.

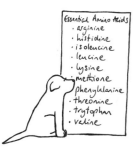

Amino acids may be divided into two groups – *essential* (or indispensable) and *non-essential* (or dispensable). Essential amino acids are those which must be present in the diet as the body is unable to synthesize them at a rate sufficient to meet the animal's requirements. The actual amino acids counted as essential varies from species to species. There are ten amino acids which are essential for the dog:

- arginine
- histidine
- isoleucine
- leucine
- lysine
- methione
- phenylalanine
- threonine
- trytophan
- valine

The cat requires the same ten amino acids plus taurine. Taurine is only obtainable from animal proteins.

Cystine and tyrosine are able to replace their precursors (methionine and phenylalanine respectively) to a certain degree in the body. In both cases the linked amino acids, methionine and cystine, and phenylalanine and tyrosine, are thought to produce a greater effect than methionine and phenylalanine alone. Cystine and tyrosine are therefore sometimes listed as essential amino acids. This is only true when the diet is deficient in their precursors.

Non-essential amino acids can be manufactured by the body from other amino acids, but their inclusion in the diet will mean that a lesser quantity of essential amino acids is required. Since cell replacement and repair is an ongoing feature of the living creature, essential amino acids need to be present in the diet on a daily basis.

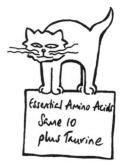

Cystine and tyrosine are only essential when diet is deficient in methionine and phenylalanine.

Sources

Proteins occur in both animals and plants, e.g. muscle meat and beans. Quality or biological value (see below) is important as the higher values will be best utilized by the body leaving few waste residues to be excreted.

Required for

- tissue building and growth, the structural components of cells
- movement by muscle contraction
- providing strength with flexibility in ligaments, tendons and cartilage

- transport (haemoglobin) and storage of oxygen in muscles (myoglobin)
- transport of other nutrients, e.g. lipids as lipoproteins.

Proteins serve as:

- enzymes – catalysts in many metabolic reactions. All enzymes are proteins.
- hormones – controlling metabolism, growth and reproduction. Not all hormones are proteins
- body protection
  (a) lubricants in mucus help prevent physical damage
  (b) innate immunity, skin, nails, claws, etc
  (c) adaptive immunity, antibodies
- an energy source.

Protein deficiency can interfere with any of the above systems, leading to poor growth or loss of body-weight, poor coat condition and impaired immunity among other problems.

If more protein is consumed than is needed for growth, repair and other functions, the excess is used for energy or stored as fat. This leaves nitrogenous wastes, which are converted to urea by the liver and excreted primarily through the kidney. Energy is produced less efficiently from protein than from fat or carbohydrate.

Biological value

The quality or biological value (BV) of a nutrient is the amount of that nutrient absorbed and utilized by the body, i.e. the difference between the amount consumed and that excreted. It is expressed as a percentage and can be applied to all nutrients, but is particularly used in reference to protein quality.

The biological value of a protein is a measure of how closely the proportions of essential amino acids match the requirements of the animal. High biological value proteins are highly digestible and leave fewer waste products to be excreted from the body. In general, animal proteins are of higher biological value than plant proteins.

A protein that contains all or most of the essential amino acids (EAAs) is a high quality protein and has a high biological value; less of it is required in the diet to meet the animal's EAAs requirements. Egg has the highest BV – 100%.

Cereal proteins are low in some amino acids, e.g. methionine and leucine, and most have a BV of less than 50%.

Definition

The biological value (BV) is a measure of the usefulness of a nutrient to an animal.

FATS (AND OILS)

Fats (solid at room temperature) and oils (liquid at room temperature) are both lipids – complex organic products which occur in two forms:

- single lipids, e.g. short- medium- and long-chain fatty acids and esters of fatty acids with glycerol, of which the triglycerides (three fatty acids plus glycerol) are most common in food
- conjugated lipids, which are lipids combined with other products, e.g. phospholipids and lipo-proteins.

Three fatty acids are referred to as essential fatty acids (EFAs):

- linoleic acid
- linolenic acid
- arachidonic acid – a major component of mamma-lian cell membranes.

The EFAs required in the diet vary between species; adult dogs can synthesize linolenic and arachidonic acids from linoleic acid, and adult cats can synthesize linolenic but not arachidonic acid.

Sources

Fats occur in both animal and plant foods, e.g. pork fat and sunflower oil. Arachidonic acid is only found in fats from animal sources.

> Arachidonic acid is only found in fats from animal sources.

Required for

- energy – major source
- storage – stores more than twice as much energy as carbohydrate for the same mass
- absorption of fat-soluble vitamins – A, D, E and K
- provision of EFAs
- formation of cell walls, thereby providing structural support
- protection of internal organs, e.g. fat pads round the kidneys
- insulation – fat layer under the skin
- waterproofing – secretions from sebaceous glands
- improved palatability of food
- manufacture of eicosanoids
- some hormones, e.g. aldosterone and prosta-glandins.

Although excess fat is a more common problem, deficiencies can also cause problems, e.g. poor coat and skin condition and reproductive failure.

Short-, medium- and long-chain fatty acids

The majority of fat in the diet is in the form of long-chain fatty acids, which contain more than 12 carbon atoms. Digestion of these requires lipase and bile salts. An emulsion of small fat droplets (micelles) is formed which increases the surface areas of the fat and ensures maximum digestion by lipase. The resultant products are absorbed by the enterocytes and attached to lipoproteins to form chylomicrons. These are released into the lacteals and then into the general circulation. Short-chain (less than eight carbon atoms) and medium-chain (eight to12 carbon atoms) are more water soluble than long-chain fatty acids. They are absorbed directly into the capillaries and transported to the liver by the hepatic portal vein. They form a useful source of calories for dogs when normal fat digestion is impaired or when lymphatic circulation from the gut fails. They should, however, be used with care, because if not absorbed they can cause discomfort and diarrhoea and are ketogenic so should not be fed to animals that are ketotic or acidotic. They should not be fed to cats as in this species they damage the liver causing hepatic lipidosis.

> Short-chain and medium-chain fatty acids are more water-soluble than long-chain.

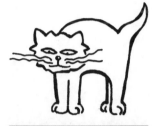

> **NB!**
> In cats, medium-chain fatty acids can damage the liver.

CARBOHYDRATES

Carbohydrates are organic compounds classified into mono-, di-, oligo- and polysaccharides:

- monosaccharides are simple sugars which are easily absorbed, e.g. glucose and fructose
- disaccharides are double sugars formed by a combination of any two monosaccharides. They are all readily hydrolysed into monosaccharides:
  e.g. glucose + glucose = maltose
  glucose + fructose = sucrose
  glucose + galactose = lactose
- oligosaccharides are short chains of monosaccharides which can be hydrolysed to simple sugars but sometimes act more like a dietary fibre
- polysaccharides are complex sugars which may be bonded in one of two ways:
  alpha-bonded polysaccharides can be split by amylase. Cooking and processing improves their digestibility, e.g. starch
  beta-bonded polysaccharides are known as 'dietary fibre' and are not digested by mammalian enzymes, e.g. cellulose.

Carbohydrate is considered a non-essential nutrient for dogs and particularly cats, as their requirements for glucose can be met by supplies of glucose precursors (amino acids and glycerol) in the diet, but the presence of carbohydrate in the diet ensures proper metabolic balance and feeding efficiency. It also spares amino acids and glycerol for their essential functions.

Sources

- cereal starch
- potatoes
- rice

Animal matter provides little or no carbohydrate.

Required for

- energy – glucose is the preferred energy source for the brain, nervous tissue and both red and white blood cells
- maintaining blood glucose levels
- producing lactose during lactation
- aids in lipid metabolism
- stored as glycogen, a readily accessible energy source, especially for muscles
- converted to and stored as fat when eaten in excess.

As carbohydrate is regarded as a non-essential component of the diet of dogs and cats, in theory deficiencies do not occur. However, dietary fibre does have a role to play in the diet of the dog (and sometimes of the cat), although less so than for humans. In these cases problems helped by fibre will be worsened without it.

> Dietary fibre plays less of a role in animal diets than for humans.

DIETARY FIBRE

Dietary fibre (or roughage) consists of those carbohydrates of plant origin which mammalian enzymes cannot digest. They may, however, be utilized by bacteria resident within the gastrointestinal tract. It is important in the diet because of its effects on motility and on the gut ecosystem.

As already mentioned, starch and fibre are similar polysaccharide chains but, while starch has its molecules linked by alpha bonds, fibre has them linked by beta bonds. Mammalian enzymes can split the alpha bonds, particularly after cooking or processing, but not beta bonds and so fibre is rendered indigestible.

The major components of dietary fibre are the carbohydrates, cellulose, hemicellulose, pectin, gums and mucilages, together with lignin (a polyphenol).

Fructo-oligosaccharides and lactulose are also included with fibre because they behave in a similar way in the gut.

Chemically (and traditionally) dietary fibre can be classified according to its solubility in water:

- soluble – pectins, gums, mucilages
- insoluble – cellulose, hemicellulose, lignin.

Alternatively, fibre may be classified biologically (and perhaps more relevantly) according to its utilization by gut bacteria:

- poorly fermentable – cellulose, oat fibre
- moderately fermentable – beet pulp, gum arabic
- highly fermentable – guar gum, fructo-oligosac-charides, lactulose.

Although dietary fibre is not classed as a nutrient and not considered an essential component of a diet, it is important and does affect the health and efficient functioning of the gastrointestinal tract in several ways:

- it delays gastric emptying
- it alters nutrient absorption, adsorption and metabolism
- it normalizes transit time through the gut
- it maintains the structural integrity of the gut mucosa
- it increases the water-holding capacity of faeces
- it adds bulk to the faeces.

Dietary fibre does have disadvantages:

- flatulence and borborygmi – particularly when large quantities are introduced suddenly into the diet
- increased faecal output.

In addition, decreased digestibility of protein, fat and carbohydrate, together with decreased uptake of some minerals, could lead to inadequate intake of these minerals under some circumstances.

In the wild, carnivores tend to eat all parts of their prey, both digestible and indigestible, so fibre can be regarded as a natural part of the diet.

VITAMINS

Vitamins are complex organic substances required in very small quantities to maintain growth, health and survival of living creatures. Plants can manufacture the vitamins they require, but animals on the whole cannot, and therefore require them as an essential part of the diet. The dietary source may be in the form of a

precursor from which the animal is able to manufacture the vitamin. Some vitamins are produced by
bacteria within the gut which may then be utilized by
the host.

There are 13 major vitamins, A, B complex (eight
vitamins), C, D, E and K and these take part in many
of the chemical reactions of metabolism.

Vitamins act as:

- enzymes
- coenzymes – molecules that attach to a protein to
  form active enzymes
- enzyme precursors.

Since most metabolic reactions are but one part of a
sequence of reactions, slowing of any one reaction
through the absence of a vitamin can have widespread
effects on the body.

A lack or poor absorption of a vitamin causes a
deficiency; an excess is known as hypervitaminosis.

Vitamins can be classified by solubility:

- fat-soluble vitamins – A, D, E and K. These are
  absorbed from the gut along with fat and can be
  stored in the body, so that a daily intake is not
  required. Over-supplementation can lead to hypervitaminosis and toxicity
- water-soluble vitamins – B complex and C. These
  are not stored in the body in significant amounts
  and excesses are excreted in urine. A daily intake is
  required and a deficiency may occur at times of
  excessive water loss, e.g. polyuria and diarrhoea or
  when gastrointestinal disorders alter microbial
  populations.

Sources of vitamins and their role in metabolism are
shown in Tables 1.1 and 1.2. Some vitamins are
actually a group of related compounds which have the
same biological activity. In these cases the name listed
is either that of the parent compound or that of the
most widely distributed compound.

Choline, required for cell membranes and neuro-
transmitters, is often listed as a B vitamin, but there is
some debate as to whether this is the case. It is present
in many plant and animal materials and mammals are
able to synthesize it within the body. It is required in
larger quantities than other vitamins.

Carnitine is another substance which is described in
some texts as a member of the B complex group, but in
others as a quasi-vitamin (vitamin-like). It is synthesized in the liver but is also required in the diet and is
found in cardiac and skeletal muscle and also in milk.
It assists in the oxidation of fatty acids and is
particularly important for those animals that obtain
most of their energy from fats, e.g. neonates and

Table 1.1 **Fat-soluble vitamins**

(Sources in parentheses are those not normally part of a cat's diet)

Vitamin	Sources	Required for
Vitamin A Retinol	Fish liver oils Liver, kidney, egg yolk. (Green vegetables and carrots contain the precursor carotene. This can be converted to vitamin A by dogs but not cats)	Visual pigments in retina. Healthy skin. Normal body growth. Correct cell division
Vitamin D D_2 ergocalciferol D_3 cholecalciferol	Synthesis by sunlight's U/V radiation in the skin or preformed in the diet, fish oils, egg yolk, dairy products	Absorption of calcium and phosphorus from gut. Maintenance of calcium and phosphorus levels in blood and bone. Tooth formation
Vitamin E α-tocopherol Destroyed by rancid fats	Liver. (Wheat germ) Level of vitamin E required is influenced by selenium – see mineral section	Antioxidant, protects lipids especially polyunsaturated fatty acids, from damage caused by free radicals formed during metabolic processes
Vitamin K Quinone-type compounds	Intestinal bacteria – may be required in diet after antibacterial treatment. (Green vegetables)	Formation of prothrombin and clotting factors

working dogs fed on an energy-dense (i.e. high-fat) diet. Extra amounts are also required in sick or convalescent animals whose energy requirements are higher than normal. Supplementation at these times may assist recovery.

Antivitamins

Antivitamins are factors within the diet which either degrade or inhibit a vitamin so that it is unavailable to the host animal and may lead to deficiency diseases. Examples of antivitamins include:

- thiaminase, which occurs in the viscera of some raw fish and degrades thiamine. It is also present in some plants, e.g. bracken
- avidin in egg whites inhibits the uptake of biotin; however, egg yolk contains high levels of biotin which eliminates the problem when whole egg is fed.

Both thiaminase and avidin are destroyed by heat.

Table 1.2 Water-soluble vitamins

(Sources in parentheses are those not normally part of a cat's diet)

Vitamin	Sources	Required for
Vitamin B_1 Thiamin – sensitive to excessive heat	Brewer's yeast, fish egg yolk. (Cereal grains, green vegetables and pulses)	Carbohydrate metabolism. Maintenance of nervous system
Vitamin B_2 Riboflavin – sensitive to light	Liver, kidneys, milk, egg. (Cereals). Some synthesis in gut	Part of various enzyme systems. Carbohydrate, fat and protein metabolism. Correct growth. Healthy skin
Pantothenic acid	Liver, kidneys, eggs. (Wheatgerm)	Carbohydrate, fat and some amino-acid metabolism. Correct antibody response
Niacin	Meats, liver, fish. (Rice, potatoes, pulses). Tryptophan can be converted to niacin by dogs but not cats	Carbohydrate, fat and protein metabolism. Healthy oral and pharyngeal tissues
Vitamin B_6 Pyridoxine	Muscle meats, eggs. (Cereal grains and vegetables)	Amino acid metabolism. Growth
Folic acid	Fish, liver, kidneys, yeast. Synthesis in gut	Nucleic acid synthesis and cell replication. Linked with B_{12} in formation of red blood cells
Biotin	Bacterial synthesis – may need dietary source after treatment. Liver, kidneys, egg yolk, milk, yeast	Gluconeogenesis. Production of energy. Normal growth. Healthy skin
Vitamin B_{12} Cobalamin – can be stored in the body	Liver, kidneys, heart	Closely linked to folic acid in formation of red blood cells. Normal functioning of nervous system. Fat and carbohydrate metabolism
Vitamin C Ascorbic acid – destroyed by heat	Normally synthesized from glucose, but dietary source recommended in stressed dogs and cats or those with hepatic disease. (Fresh fruits and vegetables)	Capillary and mucosal integrity. Wound healing

- warfarin (a dicoumarol derivative) is an anticoagulant which acts as an antivitamin, blocking the uptake of vitamin K.

MINERALS

These are inorganic substances that form the mineral component of the body. In total, minerals comprise less than 1% of bodyweight and yet are essential for correct growth and functioning of the body. They can be divided into two groups based on the amounts required by the body.

Macrominerals

The body's requirement for these is expressed in parts per hundred. 1 pph = 10 grams/kilogram diet. Minerals from this group with known dietary requirements are calcium, chlorine, magnesium, phosphorus, potassium and sodium. Their sources and roles are listed in Table 1.3. Macrominerals maintain:

- acid–base balance
- osmotic pressure, needed to maintain fluid balance
- transmembrane activity – general cellular function, nerve conduction and muscle contraction
- structural integrity.

Microminerals

The body's requirement for these is expressed in parts per million. 1 ppm = 1 milligram/kilogram diet. Minerals from this group with known dietary requirements are copper, iodine, iron, manganese, selenium and zinc. Their sources and roles are listed in Table 1.4. Microminerals are involved in the control of many diverse biological functions.

Trace elements

These are minerals acting as catalysts at cellular level, regulating many functions, including the uptake of macrominerals. The amounts required are not known but are very small and would probably be expressed in microgram/kilogram units.

Table 1.3 Macrominerals

(Sources in parentheses are those not normally part of a cat's diet)

Mineral	Sources	Required for
Calcium	Milk, eggs. (Green vegetables)	Development of bones and teeth. Blood clotting. Muscle and nerve function. Enzyme activation
Chloride	Common salt	Maintenance of osmotic pressure, acid–base and water balance
Magnesium	Meat. (Green vegetables)	Development of bones and teeth. Energy metabolism. Enzyme activation
Phosphorus	Milk, eggs, meat. (Vegetables)	Development of bones and teeth. Energy utilization. Enzyme systems. Phospholipids in cell membranes. Constituent of nucleic acids
Potassium	Meat. (Fruit and vegetables)	Nerve and muscle action. Protein synthesis. Maintenance of osmotic pressure, acid–base and water balance
Sodium	Common salt, milk, meat, eggs. (Vegetables)	Nerve and muscle action. Maintenance of osmotic pressure, acid–base and water balance

Trace elements believed to be essential for dogs and cats include chromium, cobalt, fluorine, molybdenum, nickel, silicon, sulphur and vanadium.

The role minerals play in the diet is complex. Each mineral has several functions and many functions require more than one mineral. It is generally accepted that if an animal is eating an appropriate balanced diet with a variety of ingredients, its mineral requirements will be met without any supplementation, but deficiencies may occur under certain circumstances and these may cause upsets in a wide range of metabolic reactions. Excesses can also create imbalances as some minerals compete for the same sites of absorption – too great an uptake of one may mean too little uptake of another. Some microminerals are involved in the animal's immune system and deficiencies of these result in impaired host defences.

Table 1.4 **Microminerals**

(Sources in parentheses are those not normally part of a cat's diet)

Mineral	Sources	Required for
Copper	Liver, meat, fish	Bone and haemoglobin formation. Melanin production. A constituent of many enzymes particularly those involved with protein synthesis
Iodine	Fish, shellfish	Component of growth hormone – thyroxine
Iron	Liver, meat. (Green vegetables)	Component of haemoglobin and myoglobin. Utilization of oxygen. Constituent of many enzymes
Manganese	Liver, kidneys	Enzyme activator. Growth factor in bone development. Component of connective tissue
Selenium	Meat, offal. (Cereals)	Linked with vitamin E and can replace it to some degree. A component of an enzyme – glutathione peroxidase – acting as an antioxidant
Zinc	Liver, fish, shellfish	A component of enzyme systems, particularly those linked with protein synthesis. Correct wound healing. Healthy immune system

Antioxidants

Several vitamins and minerals are listed as having antioxidant properties, but what are antioxidants and what do they do?

Antioxidants are those vitamins and minerals which, together with some enzymes, can neutralize free radicals produced as byproducts of chemical reactions necessary to sustain life, e.g. cellular respiration.

Free radicals are highly reactive and unstable molecules. Their instability is due to the presence of a single, free electron which needs a second electron to pair with and so restore the equilibrium that nature prefers. To do this the free radical takes an electron from a neighbouring molecule which is itself then rendered unstable; it in turn takes an electron from a third molecule and a chain reaction is started which damages the cell wall allowing the contents to spill out and destroying the cell.

Free radicals, when kept in check by the body's antioxidant mechanisms, have an essential role to play – they are involved in enzymatic processes and in the production of hormones. They are also instrumental in the elimination of bacteria, viruses and toxins, but problems arise when the normal balance is upset and the body's antioxidant resources are overwhelmed. Free radicals then attack cells that would normally be protected, resulting in inappropriate cell and tissue damage. The unsaturated fatty acids in the cell membrane are most affected, interfering with the transport of nutrients and waste products into and out of the cell, along with reduction of the cell's resistance to bacteria and viruses. Many age-related changes such as arthritis and heart disease are thought to be due to damage caused by oxygen free radicals.

Exposure to UV light and radiation, air pollution and residues from herbicides and pesticides in food, along with illness and the drugs that treat it, all contribute to excessive levels of free radical production. The amount of damage caused depends on the balance between free radicals and antioxidants present.

> Many age-related changes such as arthritis and heart disease are thought to be due to damage caused by oxygen free radicals.

Sources of antioxidants

Antioxidant enzyme pathways exist within the body. These are largely genetically determined and may not be able to respond adequately to excessive free radical production.

Dietary antioxidants include vitamins E, A and C and several minerals, principally selenium, but also copper, iron, manganese and zinc. These minerals are associated with antioxidant enzymes and a deficiency can interfere with the function of their related enzymes. Clearly dietary antioxidants can be varied according to need but are also dependent on the body's ability to absorb and utilize them.

Antioxidant minerals are mainly active within cells but antioxidant vitamins are able to circulate in the bloodstream and mop up any free radicals which may be present there.

Vitamin E is a potent antioxidant and is fat soluble. Its main function in the body is to protect lipid membranes, the unsaturated fatty acids, as stated earlier, being particularly sensitive to free radical activity. Immune system cells have plasma membranes which are high in polyunsaturated fatty acids and are therefore particularly susceptible to oxidative damage. These cells also normally have a higher than average vitamin E level and any deficiencies in this vitamin will have serious effects in these cells, impairing the animal's immune response.

Questions

1. How much water needs to be lost from the body before the animal becomes seriously ill?
2. Metabolic water supplies around 10% of the animal's daily water requirement. Where does this come from?
3. Essential amino acids need not be present in the diet on a daily basis. True or false?
4. Taurine is available from both animal and plant sources. True or false?
5. What is an enzyme?
6. Name the three essential fatty acids.
7. What are oligosaccharides?
8. Avidin is an antivitamin. It inhibits the uptake of which vitamin?
9. Macrominerals are measured in parts per _____ . Microminerals are measured in parts per _____.
10. What is the purpose of antioxidants?

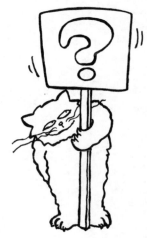

② Energy

INTRODUCTION

In the list of essential requirements for animals, energy comes third after oxygen and water. Animals, unlike humans, eat chiefly to satisfy their energy needs, so in order to know how much to feed, we need to plunge headlong into the maze of abbreviations, complex equations and technical terms that surround energy.

To recap

Essential requirements:

1 Oxygen
2 Water
3 Energy

WHAT IS ENERGY?

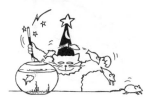

The magic of energy

Energy is the power driving all functions of the living creature. Inanimate objects contain energy, but are unable to prevent its loss, neither are they able to replace it.

Energy assumes several forms, e.g. heat, mechanical or chemical energy. It cannot be created or destroyed but may be changed from one form to another. Animals (and humans) consume energy in chemical form via energy-containing nutrients, and metabolism within each individual cell converts this chemical energy into new forms as required. In these reactions, part of the energy is converted to heat, some of which is required to maintain body temperature but much of it is 'lost' from the body, thus requiring fresh supplies of chemical energy to be consumed.

Energy can be measured either as joules (a measure of work done) or as calories, one calorie being equal to 4.184 joules. One calorie is the amount of heat required to raise one gram of water through one degree Celsius. The kilocalorie, kcal or Calorie (with a capital C) is equal to 1000 calories and is the unit that anyone who has tried to diet will be familiar with.

All animals use energy all of the time, but their exact requirements depend on many factors, e.g. age, level of activity, physiological status and size (partic-

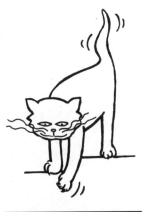

Definition

One calorie is the amount of heat required to raise one gram of water through one degree Celsius.

ularly in relation to surface area). Just as the driver of a car in city streets requires his vehicle to travel at a different rate to that required when travelling down a clear motorway, so the body requires its metabolism to proceed at different rates at different times.

An animal's daily energy requirement (DER) is composed of several fractions:

- Basal energy requirement (BER), or basal metabolic rate (BMR) or basal energy expenditure (BEE). All these terms represent the amount of energy required to keep vital organs functioning continuously, e.g. breathing, circulation, kidney function, brain activity and temperature control. It assumes that the animal is completely inactive some 12 hours after a meal and in a stress-free, thermoneutral environment. Attempting to measure BER is impractical as the resultant stress for the animal raises its metabolic rate and hence its energy usage.
- Resting energy rate (RER). This represents the energy required by a relaxed animal in a thermoneutral environment 12 hours after eating. Although it has been calculated that RER may be 1.25 × BER, they are usually very similar and the two are often regarded as interchangeable values.
- Maintenance energy requirement (MER). This represents RER plus the energy needed for exercise, digestion and absorption of food. Average values for this are:
  – dog RER × 2
  – cat RER × 1.4.

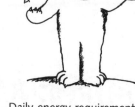

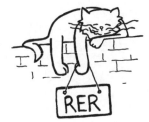

Daily energy requirements

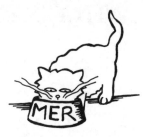

CALCULATING ENERGY REQUIREMENTS

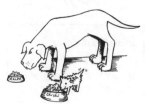

Size matters!

The relationship between size and energy requirements is not straightforward. It is based on the interaction between the animal's weight and surface area. This is because one of the main routes for energy loss from the body is in the form of heat, chiefly through radiation and convection from the body surfaces. It follows that the larger the surface area in relation to the bulk of the body, the higher is the heat loss and the greater the need for energy replacement. A Chihuahua with a large surface area to bodyweight ratio requires more energy per kilogram than a Great Dane with a low surface area to bodyweight ratio.

Several complicated formulae to calculate RER exist to enthral all mathematicians among you and seriously confuse the rest. Thankfully a simpler one has been devised for animals weighing more than 2 kilograms and is shown in Table 2.1.

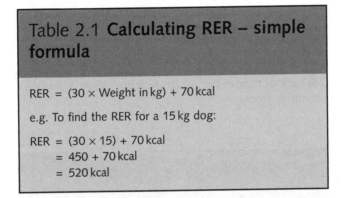

Table 2.1 Calculating RER – simple formula

RER = (30 × Weight in kg) + 70 kcal

e.g. To find the RER for a 15 kg dog:

RER = (30 × 15) + 70 kcal
    = 450 + 70 kcal
    = 520 kcal

Sadly, as weight decreases, this 'simple' formula becomes increasingly less accurate, so for those of you who insist on knowing the energy requirements of a small animal, a more complex equation needs to be used. Table 2.2 shows the one generally accepted for use in dogs and cats – the use of a calculator is actively encouraged.

Table 2.2 Calculating RER – complex formula

RER = 70 × (Weight in $kg^{0.75}$)

e.g. To find the RER for a pup weighing 500 g:

Remember to convert grams to kilograms.

500 g = 0.5 kg
RER = 70 × ($0.5^{0.75}$)
($0.5^{0.75}$) is found by taking the square root of 0.5 twice and then cubing the result:

$\sqrt{0.5}$ = 0.707

$\sqrt{0.707}$ = 0.841

0.841 × 0.841 × 0.841 = 0.595.

RER = 70 × 0.595 kcal
    = 41.65 kcal

(Based on the simple formula, RER would be 85 kcal – more than double the true requirement.)

ENERGY REQUIREMENTS IN SICKNESS

Sick and injured animals have altered energy requirements, but the calculations for ill animals are based on the RER as it is assumed that they will be inactive and often confined in a small area. Surgery, trauma and sepsis, etc., all increase the animal's energy requirements but, again, this is based on the RER figure. Table 2.3 lists the factors used to multiply RER in varying circumstances.

Table 2.3 Energy requirements in sickness

Burns: moderate	RER × 1.5
severe	RER × 2.0
Cage rest	RER × 1.25
Cancer: early	RER × 1.25
late	RER × 1.75
Sepsis	RER × 1.5
Surgery/trauma: mild	RER × 1.25
severe	RER × 1.5

ENERGY REQUIREMENTS IN HEALTH

As we have seen, the 'average dog on the street' – a normal healthy pet – will have a MER of RER × 2, but inactive dogs (e.g. the ones left at home sleeping all day) will require less energy and working dogs will require more. Growth, pregnancy and lactation also affect the daily energy requirement. Low environmental temperatures increase the need for energy but somewhat surprisingly, higher than average environmental temperatures increase the requirement further. The animal has to work harder to lose heat than gain it. Table 2.4 lists the appropriate factors by which MER should be multiplied in these cases.

Table 2.4 **Energy requirements in health**

Growth (dogs) weaning to	50% adult weight	MER × 2
	50–80% adult weight	MER × 1.5
	80–100% adult weight	MER × 1.2
(cats)	less than 3 months	MER × 2.5
	3–5 months	MER × 1.6
	5–7 months	MER × 1.2
Gestation (dogs)	1st third	MER × 1.0
	2nd third	MER × 1.1
	last third	MER × 1.2–1.3
(cats)	1st third	MER × 1.1
	2nd third	MER × 1.2
	last third	MER × 1.2–1.3
Peak lactation		MER × 2–4 depending on size of litter
Inactivity		MER × 0.8
Cold		MER × 1.25–1.75
Tropical heat, up to		MER × 2.5

All figures are estimates. Each animal is an individual and should be treated as such.

ENERGY CONTENT OF A FOOD

Anyone who has ever dieted will know that different foods contain different amounts of calories (energy). The term 'energy density' refers to this energy content per unit of weight, usually shown as 'kcal per 100 g'. A food needs to have an energy density that is sufficient to provide for an animal's calorific needs contained in an amount that the animal has the physical capacity to eat. If a food has too low an energy density, the animal will be unable to consume enough of it to meet its energy needs. If the energy density is too high, then the animal is liable to over-consume on calories and become overweight, or if the animal stops eating when its calorific needs are met, the body's requirements for other nutrients may not be met.

Foods with a high energy content are referred to as 'energy dense'. Puppies and kittens have high energy needs but very small stomachs so need energy-dense foods.

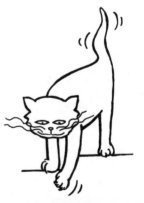

Definition

Energy density = the number of kcal per 100 g of food.

The gross energy (GE), is the total energy content of a food and is measured in a calorimeter. A weighed quantity of the food is burnt in the calorimeter and the heat (energy) that is given off represents the gross energy. When a food is ingested, not all the energy contained in it is available for use by the animal. The digestibility of any nutrient is a measure of the difference between the amount eaten and the amount lost through the faeces, so:

- Gross energy – Faecal energy = Digestible energy

Increasing digestibility tends to reduce faecal quantity and reduce demands on those body systems designed to eliminate waste.

Further amounts of energy are lost through urine and the portion left is known as metabolizable energy (ME), in effect the usable energy.

- Digestible energy – Urinary losses = Metabolizable energy

Part of this usable energy is converted to heat during digestion and absorption and although some will be used to maintain body temperature, more of it will be 'lost' to the animal.

- Metabolizable energy – Heat increment = Net energy

Net energy is available to the animal for upkeep of vital functions, physical activity, growth and repair of tissue, and adaptation to changing environments, both internal and external. Net energy is used primarily for maintenance and then for production (e.g. growth, reproduction and physical activity). If there is insufficient energy left after maintenance needs are satisfied, production will not take place.

Figure. 2.1 summarizes the above.

Quoted calorie values of foods are the calories available to the animal to be used as physiological fuel, i.e. metabolizable energy. These calorie values are variously quoted as carbohydrate and protein, 3.5 or 3.8 kcal/g, and fat as 8.5, 8.7 or 8.9 kcal/g. For ease of calculation they are often taken as:

- protein 4 kcal/g
- carbohydrate 4 kcal/g
- fat 9 kcal/g.

PALATABILITY AND ACCEPTABILITY

Although animals mainly eat to satisfy their energy requirements, palatability and acceptability are also factors to be considered.

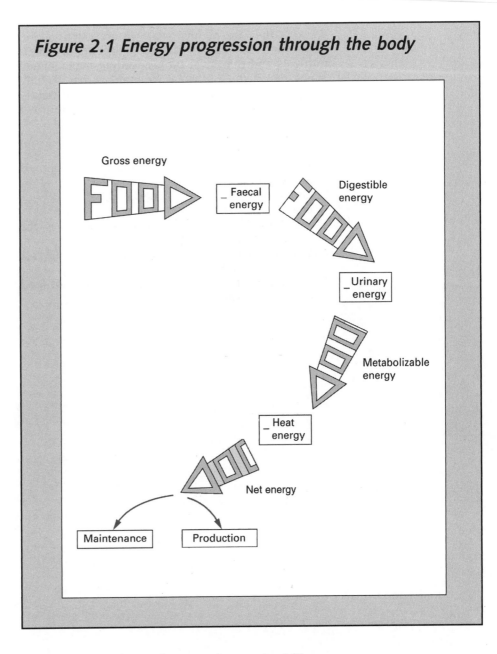

Figure 2.1 Energy progression through the body

Gross energy

− Faecal energy

Digestible energy

− Urinary energy

Metabolizable energy

− Heat energy

Net energy

Maintenance

Production

Palatability indicates how much an animal likes a food. It is an objective value as different animals have preferences for different foods. It can be affected by temperature (warm food smells stronger and more attractive), by salt or fat content (both tend to increase palatability) and by its texture (how it feels in the mouth. Again different animals have different preferences).

Acceptability considers whether enough of a food will be eaten to meet the animal's energy requirements.

Foods that are highly palatable are often calorie dense and can lead to the consumption of excess nutrients and calories if proper feeding management is not exercised – a fact that we humans may be only too aware of. A food need only be sufficiently palatable to ensure adequate energy and nutrient intake, i.e. acceptability.

Questions
1. Energy requirements for sick and injured animals are based on the _____ energy rate.
2. Gross energy – _____ energy = _____ energy.
3. The 'usable' energy of a food is known as the _____ energy.
4. Why are energy-dense foods recommended for puppies and kittens?
5. Name three factors that affect the amount of food eaten by an animal.

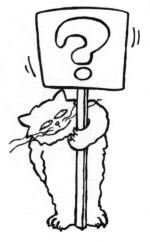

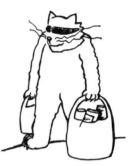

③ Types of food

INTRODUCTION

Time was when dogs were fed household scraps, with bones from the butcher if they were lucky. Cats were given a saucer of milk, fish skins and fish heads when available and caught mice, birds, etc., to supply the rest of their needs.

Nowadays things are rather different. A large proportion of pets receive most of their dietary requirements from commercial petfoods. There are still those owners who, for a variety of reasons, prefer to feed home-made diets and the veterinary nurse should be able to give advice on these when required to do so.

Increasing knowledge constantly refines the nutritionalist view of an ideal diet and it becomes more and more difficult to provide this ideal diet without the manipulation made possible by technology. Having said that, pets requiring special diets, e.g. low-protein or low-fat diets, may prefer home-made to commercial varieties (suitable recipes for such occasions are available from some of the major pet food manufacturers) and a food that is eaten, even if not the ideal, is better than the ideal diet which is left in the bowl.

Diets, then, fall into two categories, home-made and proprietary diets.

HOME-MADE DIETS

It is stating the obvious to say that in the wild, animals eat raw, unprocessed food, but it is a fact that is often overlooked. They eat not only what is, to humans, the acceptable bits, muscle meats, liver and kidney, but also those we consider unacceptable, bones, brain, skin, gut and gut contents, thus giving a much more balanced diet. We are probably not going to feed whole carcasses, but feeding raw meat and bone does form a more natural diet, even though many people will have concerns about giving bones to dogs.

Problems seen in veterinary surgeries caused by feeding bones range from pieces of bone stuck in the mouth through damaged gut to constipation. Cooked bones are more brittle and more likely to cause problems, but even the large uncooked 'knuckle' bones have been known to initiate a sudden visit to the vet. We do, however, only see the problem cases and there may be many dogs that are regularly given bones without any problems arising. Many scavenging dogs, for example, will regularly eat chicken carcasses, chop bones, etc., with impunity. The best approach is to warn owners of the potential risks so they can make an informed decision, to feed or not to feed bones!

Cooking alters foodstuffs; cereals and vegetables become easier to digest because starches in them are broken down, but some nutrients are destroyed by heat and overheating proteins can lead to chemical reactions taking place, which make them less digestible. Taking this into account, home-made diets should only be lightly cooked and any water used in cooking should be kept and mixed with the food, thus saving leached nutrients. Salt should not be added. Home-made diets should also contain as much variety as possible to ensure adequate nutrition. It is when trying to formulate home-made diets that the preceding energy calculations come into their own.

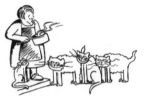

Great! Another culinary disaster

It is important to stress to owners that cats are obligate carnivores whose bodies are programmed to function on a diet consisting mainly of protein and fat. They normally eat little carbohydrate other than that in the gut of their prey. Proprietary cat foods now seem to contain increased amounts of carbohydrate, leading owners to think that this is acceptable practice. Commercially prepared foods are supplemented with the necessary nutrients, e.g. taurine, which are of animal origin to ensure an adequate supply. This supplementation is normally not possible with home-made diets and those which contain too much carbohydrate will have inadequate supplies of some nutrients. Cats cannot be vegetarians. Table 3.1 lists foods suitable for inclusion in home-made diets.

Providing a balanced home-made diet is possible, but requires considerable skill, can be expensive, and cooking may produce smells which are unacceptable to human noses but will cause a queue of the neighbourhood's cats to form on the doorstep. For these and other reasons, the majority of people will opt for those foods which are specially prepared, ready to feed and readily available – proprietary diets.

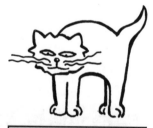

NB!
Cats cannot be vegetarians

Table 3.1 Sources of nutrients for home-made diets

Protein
Meat – trim fat (may be excessive amounts otherwise)
Fish
Eggs and cheese
Milk powder (small amounts)
Pulses – beans and peas (beware low palatability and tendency to cause flatulence)

Fats and oils
Animal or vegetable origin (use sparingly, fat is energy dense, high fat content may reduce intake of other nutrients)

Carbohydrate
Bread and potato (also contain small amounts of protein)
Rice and pasta (easily digested)

Vitamins and minerals
Green and root vegetables are a cheap source of vitamins, minerals and fibre but low palatability, not accepted by all animals
Variety in diet will ensure adequate supply of most vitamins and minerals; use supplement if insufficient variety
Avoid over-cooking and preserve cooking water; do not add salt unless specifically advised to

PROPRIETARY DIETS

All proprietary foods are processed and therefore suffer from a degree of nutrient destruction, but manufacturers take this into account when formulating the recipes. Proprietary foods are available in a bewildering variety, but all fall into one of two categories – complete or complementary.

- Complete foods, as the name suggests, provide a complete, balanced and adequate diet when fed alone. They contain all the essential ingredients in the correct ratio to each other and to the energy content of the food.
- Complementary foods are nutritionally unbalanced and require the addition of another food to form a balanced and adequate diet. Treats are often described as complementary as it is not intended that the animal should be fed on these alone.

Whether complete or complementary, foods can also be divided into three groups – moist, semi-moist and dry.

- Moist foods contain 70–85% moisture and are available in a variety of packaging, of which the can is the most common. These products are generally preserved by heat treatment, although some meats are available frozen. Premium moist foods are usually highly palatable and can lead to obesity because the degree of palatability overrides the animal's instinct to eat only to satisfy its energy requirements. Owners perceive that their pet 'prefers' these products and so tend to feed more and exacerbate the problem.

  High protein intake means that larger amounts of the end products of protein metabolism have to be excreted, which poses problems when the animal has an existing liver or kidney problem.

  Moist foods tend to be more palatable and digestible than dry ones. They often provide more fat per unit of dry matter and are more expensive than dry foods. They require refrigeration after opening and food left in bowls tends to dry or 'go off' if not eaten immediately. The potential for food to be wasted is high.

- Semi-moist foods contain around 30% moisture. They are mostly complete foods and usually available in foil or cellophane packages. Meat and cereal ingredients are cooked and formed into a paste which is passed through an extruder and shaped into small pieces. Acids are added, lowering the pH and inhibiting the growth of bacteria and fungi. They are coated with corn (or other) syrup which binds with the water thus preventing the food from drying out and ensures that the moisture is unavailable for the growth of microorganisms. Semi-moist foods have a fairly long shelf life, they do not require refrigeration and can be fed free-choice. They are less expensive than moist foods and contain a variety of ingredients.

  The coating of syrup tends to increase the energy digestibility of the food and also makes them unsuitable for diabetic animals.

- Dry foods contain 10–14% moisture and rely on this low moisture content for their preservation. They are usually packed in bags or cardboard and divide into two groups – dry meals and biscuits. They may be complete or complementary.

  Meal types contain dry, flaked or crushed cereals and vegetables and, in some cases, dry protein concentrates. They are either packed as a mix of prepared dried ingredients or are mixed to a paste and extruded in the same way as semi-moist foods. The heat produced during extrusion ensures that starches are adequately broken down for correct digestion. The extruded shapes are then dried, sometimes coated with fat, and packaged.

The loose mix type may be less easily digested and the animal will require more to ensure adequate nutrition, providing extra work for the digestive system and more faeces for the owner to clean up. They have the advantage of visible ingredient variety, but the variation in size and weight of the ingredients causes separation, with the heavier pieces sinking to the bottom of the container. This may lead to an unbalanced diet being fed from day to day. These mixes often need soaking before feeding and if not eaten straightaway will form a rather unsavoury solid mass in the dish and may be thrown away, wasted.

Extruded foods are usually fed dry and so can be fed free-choice. They are now available as a mix of shapes and colours to provide the visual variety, which is purely a human criterion. The slightly abrasive effect of extruded foods on the teeth helps prevent the accumulation of plaque.

Biscuits are made from wheat flour and often fortified with calcium and fat-soluble vitamins. They can be shaped and cooked, or baked in large sheets which are broken into small pieces (kibble) after baking. Biscuits are complementary foods.

Dry foods are less expensive than moist or semi-moist foods. They require less storage space and do not need refrigeration, but may be less palatable than other foods.

The most expensive foods are usually 'fixed formula' foods, i.e. they contain the same raw ingredients in the same quantities in each batch manufactured. In other foods, the raw ingredients may vary from batch to batch. The overall percentage of a nutrient will remain the same but may be from a different source; this enables costs to be kept down because the raw material which is cheapest at any one time can be used.

LABELLING OF PROPRIETARY FOODS

In Britain the information carried on pet food packaging is controlled by the Trades Descriptions Act, Weights and Measures, the Feedingstuffs Regulations and some EU directives.

A Statutory Statement must be printed on every label which must be 'visible, legible, indelible and separate from other information' and must include:

- Description and directions – the type of food (complete or complementary), the species of animal for which it is intended and directions for use
- Ingredients list – the ingredients are listed in descending order, i.e. the product that is listed first, occurs in the greatest quantity. Ingredients may be listed either using category names (e.g. meat and animal derivatives) or by individual names (e.g. chicken or beef)
- Typical analysis – the percentages of protein, oil (or fat), fibre and ash, together with the percentage of moisture where this is higher than 14%
- Vitamins – where vitamins A, D or E are added, this must be declared and the level present listed (including the quantity occurring naturally in the raw materials)
- Additives – where preservatives, antioxidants or colours have been added, they must be listed using either chemical or category names
- A best-before date – the month and year must be given, the day is optional (in some cases the date order shown is month, day, year). If the actual date is printed outside the statement, its whereabouts must be stated within the Statutory Statement
- Batch number – this also can be listed elsewhere, but its whereabouts should be noted within the Statutory Statement. The date of manufacture may be used as a batch number, in which case the day, month and year are required

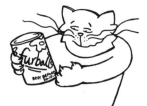

Vintage '67?

The label should also list the name and address of the company responsible for that product; this may be the manufacturer, the packer, importer, seller or distributor.

Both the Feedingstuffs Regulations and the Weights and Measures Act require the net weight of the product to be shown. The Trades Description Act requires the information given to be truthful and not misleading.

Labelling of foods which have a clinical application, i.e. a dietetic pet food, is further required to show:

- the particular purpose and species for which it is designed
- the type and level of nutrients, additives and characteristics which fit it for this purpose
- the length of time for which it should be fed. (It is assumed that dietetic foods are only for temporary use, although many of them are suitable for long-term adult maintenance.)

COMPARISONS BETWEEN DIFFERENT FOODS

The proportions of ingredients used in foods will vary, not only between manufacturers, but also between brands produced by any one manufacturer.

The typical analysis required as part of the Statutory Statement is based on the whole contents of the tin or packet, including water. This moisture content has an effect on the rest of the ingredients, drier foods being more concentrated than moist ones, so direct comparisons of nutrient content using the typical analysis are inaccurate. More accurate comparisons are obtained using a dry weight basis, i.e. comparing the ingredients of that portion of the food that is left after the moisture is removed. Table 3.2 shows the comparison between two foods, one moist and one dry (the figures shown were chosen for ease of comparison rather than an accurate reflection of the typical contents of a moist and dry food). Figure 3.1 shows a visual representation of this comparison. Similar comparisons can be drawn up for proprietary brands, which may help to explain the apparent discrepancies to owners.

Table 3.2 Comparison between moist and dry foods on a dry matter basis

Food A (tinned food) has 80% moisture, Food B (dry food) has 20% moisture, both foods contain 10% protein.

Step 1. Calculate the proportion of dry matter in each food.
Food A with 80% moisture has (100 – 80) 20% dry matter.
Food B with 20% moisture has (100 – 20) 80% dry matter.

Step 2. Calculate the protein content as a proportion of the dry matter.
Food A has a protein content of 10%, dry matter 20%
so protein content = 10/20 × 100 = 50%
Food B has a protein content of 10%, dry matter 80%
so protein content = 10/80 × 100 = 12.5%
Food A actually contains four times as much protein as Food B.

An even more accurate comparison is that based on energy content, but as most British pet food products do not give this information, we have to rely on the dry matter comparisons.

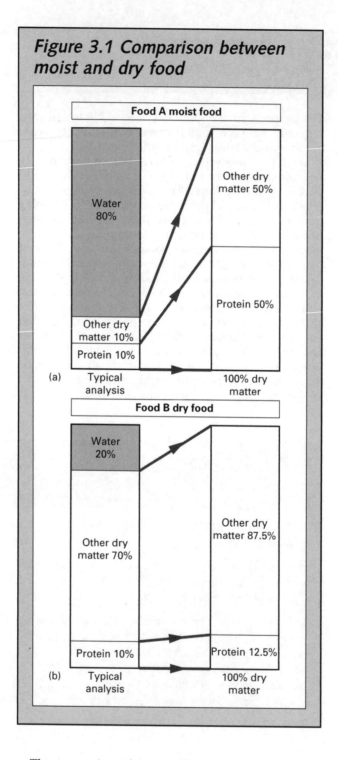

Figure 3.1 Comparison between moist and dry food

Food A moist food

Water 80%

Other dry matter 10%

Protein 10%

Other dry matter 50%

Protein 50%

(a)   Typical analysis

100% dry matter

Food B dry food

Water 20%

Other dry matter 70%

Protein 10%

Other dry matter 87.5%

Protein 12.5%

(b)   Typical analysis

100% dry matter

The comparison shown in Figure 3.1 also illustrates the difference in amounts of dry and moist foods eaten. To consume the same amount of protein, fat and other nutrients, the animal needs to eat less weight of dry food than moist food, but animals eating dry food need to drink more water to compensate for the differences in moisture content.

Cat owners will often remark that their pet drinks very little. If the cat is fed on moist foods, it may receive almost all of its daily water requirement from the food but, if the cat is then changed to a dry food, it will need to drink to satisfy its water requirements and the owner may be concerned about the sudden increase in drinking. Dogs will demonstrate a similar increase in drinking when changed to a dry food, but this seems to be less noticeable to the owners.

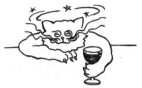

VARIETY

Variety in a pet's diet is of great importance to the owner; it may be less important to the pet. There are two schools of thought regarding the provision of variety.

The first states that given a complete, balanced diet appropriate to the age and physiological state of the animal, that diet should be fed and nothing else. Dogs and cats have no requirement for change and variety in their diet. This is a concept that many owners will find difficult to accept – not surprising when you remember the psychological associations that food has for humans. Most owners would rapidly become bored with their diet if they had to eat the same food each day and they assume that their pets feel the same way.

The second view states that variety is good for animals, that in the wild they would eat different foods according to season and circumstance, and that being used to different foods, tastes and textures, makes easier the introduction of new diets should they become medically necessary in later life.

Whichever view you subscribe to, there is some justification for saying that animals fed one food, either because they demonstrate a liking for that food, or for economic reasons on the part of the owner, will develop a preference for that food through habit. In these cases it can be difficult to introduce new foods.

As always, veterinary nurses need to consider not just what is best for the animal, but also what is acceptable to the owner. Fortunately, as some animals do have food preferences and variety is important to owners, pet food manufacturers in many cases now formulate a basic recipe and then produce it in different flavours.

A note of caution should be sounded here, as different flavours may in fact be precisely that. In some cases a common mix is made up and then different portions flavoured with lamb, beef, chicken, etc., rather like a batch of icing which can be split into different portions and coloured by the addition of different concentrates. Always read the label, especially when food sensitivities are involved.

SUPPLEMENTS

Supplements are sometimes regarded by owners as an essential part of their pet's diet, so may reasonably discussed here.

Mention of supplements is usually taken to mean the addition of vitamins and/or minerals to the animal's diet in either tablet, liquid or powder form. In the past, when balanced, lifestage foods were not available, there may well have been a need for such supplements. Nowadays it is generally accepted that a normal, healthy animal fed a balanced diet, appropriate to its age, lifestyle and species, will receive adequate amounts of vitamins and minerals.

These nutrients are needed in very small quantities and more is not necessarily better. An example is that of large breed pups being given mineral supplements to encourage bone growth. Rapid growth in these breeds is now known to be undesirable, increasing the likelihood of skeletal disorders developing.

Recommended daily amounts (RDAs) are, however, only averages and cannot take into account the quirks of the individual; certain dogs and cats with specific clinical problems may require supplementation. This should only be provided on the advice of the veterinary surgeon and the effects should be carefully monitored.

In contrast, many of the exotic species should routinely be given vitamin and mineral supplements because of the inadequacies of their diets and the artificial conditions under which they live.

Having said all that, nutritional science is a dynamic subject and research may modify present-day RDAs as, for example, in the case of antioxidants. Levels of free radicals appear to be rising in many animals, possibly due to increasing pollution levels. Current RDAs for antioxidants are probably inadequate given these increases and future recommendations may suggest higher levels than are presently included in diets.

Other dietary supplements are available for specific problems, e.g. joint and skin problems, and their use

> Many of the exotic species should routinely be given vitamin and mineral supplements because of the inadequacies of their diets and the artificial conditions under which they live.

> Dietary supplements are available for specific problems and their use can reduce or replace the need for drug therapy.

can reduce or replace the need for drug therapy in these conditions. Undoubtedly, as interest grows in these products, the number of products available and their range of applications will increase rapidly.

Questions
1. Home-made diets should be fed raw or _____ cooked, have no ____ added and contain as much _____ as possible to ensure _____ nutrition.
2. Proprietary foods are divided into two categories: _____ and _____. Which of these may be fed alone?
3. Semi-moist foods are often coated with a substance that makes them unsuitable for feeding to animals with diabetes mellitus. What is this substance?
4. An animal changing from a canned diet to a dry diet will have an apparent increase in thirst. True or false?
5. Foods should be compared on a '____ _____' or _____ _____ basis.

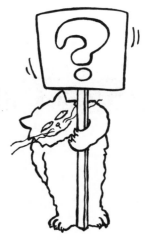

Feeding dogs and cats

FEEDING RECOMMENDATIONS

It should be stressed that the feeding guides included on pet food labels are for guidance only. The recommended amounts are based on the average energy requirements for the bodyweight given; but an average is just that – an average. Some individuals will require less, some will require more and each individual will require different amounts at different times depending on variants such as their level of exercise. Older animals will have different energy requirements than in their younger days, either because of decreased exercise or because of a natural reduction in lean body mass as a consequence of ageing. Such reductions lead to a decreased energy requirement per unit of bodyweight, even when the animal's weight remains the same as in earlier years.

Deciding how much to feed can be a matter of trial and error. Unless the animal concerned is particularly active, it is better to start with less than the recommended amount and build up the quantities if necessary. Starting with the recommended amount may lead to weight gain, which is always more difficult to correct. Body condition is the best guide as to whether the animal is being fed at the correct levels.

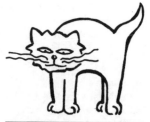

NB!
Feeding instructions included on pet food labels are for guidance only and not absolute quantities.

BODY CONDITION SCORE

It is sometimes difficult to determine what an animal's ideal weight should be. It is often said to be that of the dog or cat at one year old, and recording the animal's weight at the time of its first booster gives a baseline for future reference. There are, of course, exceptions to this generalization. For dogs and cats overfed as pups and kittens, the weight at one year is likely to be excessive and large or giant breed dogs

Figure 4.1 Body condition scoring (dogs)

(a) *Emaciated*: Obvious loss of muscle mass, no fat cover, ribs and pelvic bones easily seen

(b) *Thin*: Waist and abdominal tuck clearly present, ribs seen, pelvic bones have little tissue cover

(c) *Ideal*: Waist and abdominal tuck present, ribs can be felt but not seen

(d) *Overweight*: Waist absent, abdominal tuck disappearing, ribs felt with difficulty, fat pads forming at base of tail

(e) *Obese*: Bulges in place of waist and abdominal tuck, ribs are no longer palpable, thick fat deposits at base of tail

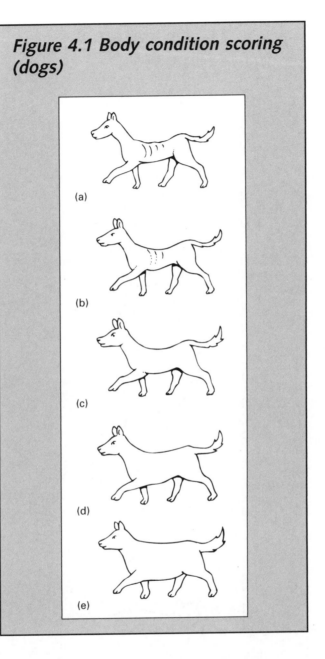

(a)

(b)

(c)

(d)

(e)

will not reach their mature weight until they are 18 months old or later. Even within a breed there will be variations in 'frame size' and it is particularly difficult to establish an ideal weight for mixed breed dogs.

Body condition scoring is a visual assessment of an animal's nutritional status, comparing the animal's shape with an ideal shape and indicating whether that animal is under- or overweight. It is somewhat subjective, particularly in dogs where breed shapes

Figure 4.2 Body condition scoring (cats)

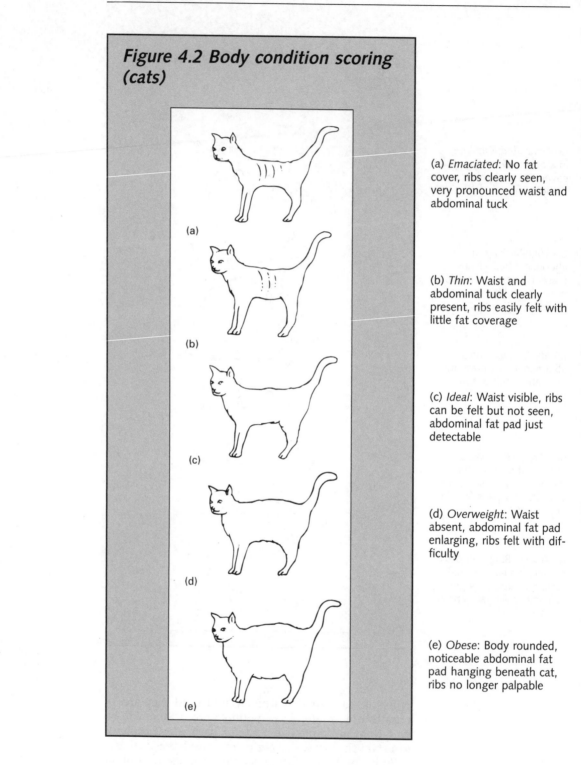

(a) *Emaciated*: No fat cover, ribs clearly seen, very pronounced waist and abdominal tuck

(b) *Thin*: Waist and abdominal tuck clearly present, ribs easily felt with little fat coverage

(c) *Ideal*: Waist visible, ribs can be felt but not seen, abdominal fat pad just detectable

(d) *Overweight*: Waist absent, abdominal fat pad enlarging, ribs felt with difficulty

(e) *Obese*: Body rounded, noticeable abdominal fat pad hanging beneath cat, ribs no longer palpable

vary a great deal, but it is a useful tool in describing to owners the concept of ideal weight. Visual prompts –'Your dog should have a waist when viewed from

Figure 4.3 Body condition scoring (rabbits)

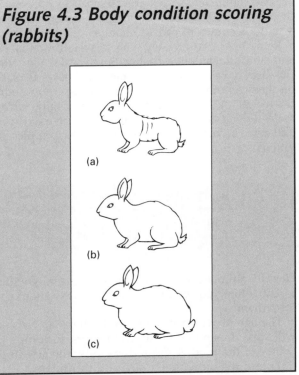

(a) *Thin*: Loss of muscle, no fat cover, ribs and other bones clearly visible

(b) *Ideal*: Correct rabbit shape, ribs felt but not seen, no abdominal bulge

(c) *Obese*: Pronounced fat layers, rounded shape, ribs no longer palpable

above' – are easier to understand and accept than relatively abstract statements –'Your dog needs to lose 'x' kilos'.

The body condition score consists of five or nine groups. For general purposes five divisions are sufficient, ranging from emaciated to obese. These groups are illustrated in Figures 4.1 (dogs) and 4.2 (cats). Condition scoring for rabbits is less well established and for these animals perhaps three groups will suffice – thin, ideal weight and obese. These are illustrated in Figure 4.3.

Owners may wish to measure their animals in addition to, or instead of, weighing them. Despite the different sites of fat deposition in dogs and cats, in both species the pelvic circumference is the measurement most likely to change with weight loss or gain. Measurements are taken with the animal in a standing position and the tape passed round the body immediately in front of the hind legs. The tape should be drawn sufficiently tight to just compress the coat against the skin. This can be a helpful visual reminder, but its reliability is questionable for a variety of reasons. It is difficult to ensure that the tape is always in exactly the same place and the same amount of pressure applied, so small changes may be

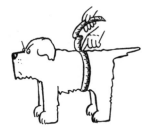

of little significance. Cats are usually less cooperative than dogs. On balance, weighing is quicker, easier and a more accurate record of change.

Remember that an easy way to weigh rabbits, cats and small dogs is in a basket. Some scales will allow the display to be set to zero once the basket is placed on them; in other cases it will be necessary to deduct the weight of the basket from the total. Digital kitchen scales which are graduated in grams are easy to use and more accurate for most small furries, puppies and kittens.

FEEDING THE HEALTHY DOG AND CAT

Healthy animals, unlike sick ones, are usually willing to eat (often too willing), but how often should we feed them?

The age at which puppies and kittens are weaned will vary, depending on several factors, including the ability of the mother to produce milk, the size of the litter and the individual's size and thriftiness. Consequently, the age at which puppies and kittens move to their new homes will vary.

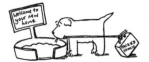

Regardless of age, the complete change of environment, linked with loss of mother and siblings, places enormous stress on these tiny animals. Change in diet and feeding regime at this point only adds to the stress, pushing many over their stress threshold and leading to digestive upsets. If at all possible, the original food(s) and timing of meals should be adhered to for the first few days, after which the new owner may gradually change to the food(s) and regime that he or she prefers.

Puppies and kittens have very small stomachs so need feeding little and often. Generally speaking, the younger the animal at weaning, the smaller and more frequent should be the meals. As they grow, their stomach capacity increases and frequency of feeding can decrease. A good plan to follow in the early stages is to provide food for a period of 10–20 minutes, removing what is left at the end of that time and offering fresh food at the next meal time. When pups and kittens move to their new homes they will probably be on four meals a day. As they grow they will gradually show less interest in one meal; this can then be dropped and the intervals between the remaining three increased. Similarly, in time, one of these three meals is likely to become less popular and the growing animal can be reduced to two meals per day. There are, of course, always exceptions to rules, and some animals will continue to eat whenever food is put before them. In these cases the owner will have to exercise restraint on the animal's behalf if obesity is not to follow. While skinny youngsters clearly need extra care, the 'roly-poly pup' image should never be considered the ideal puppy shape.

When the animal reaches adulthood, it is worth thinking about how dogs and cats feed in the wild. Despite their many thousands of years of domestication, basic traits still prevail, perhaps not too surprising considering that until the middle of the twentieth century, proprietary pet foods were not readily available and most pets still had to fend for themselves to a large degree.

Most cats tend to be 'snackers'. This reflects their natural feeding pattern – expend energy catching mouse, eat small meal, sleep to recover, expend energy catching another mouse/bird, etc. Dogs tend to act as scavengers – find carrion, eat as much as possible because who knows when the next meal will appear, or hunting as a pack – eat as much as possible before someone else pushes me out. In the wild, they will also snack between meals on small animals, fruits, etc. – sounds familiar?

Although a generalization, this does go some way to explaining the difference in feeding habits of the two species and indicates that limited mealtimes are best for dogs and food left permanently available for cats, which are usually much better at regulating appetite. (The amount on offer should be measured out at the beginning of the day to guard against obesity in those cats which are not quite so good at regulating their appetites or where high palatability is likely to override satiety factors.) These systems break down in multi-pet households where the top cat will eat more than its fair share and dogs empty all bowls in one sitting on the 'just in case' principle. Competition also seems to encourage overeating.

The two examples above illustrate the two main methods of feeding:

- meal feeding (dogs) and
- ad lib (cats).

Meal feeding can be subdivided into time-restricted feeding and food-restricted feeding. The former provides an unrestricted amount of food for a restricted time, after which period the remaining food (if any) is removed. This may encourage the animal to gulp the food down in order to eat as much as possible in the given time. The latter supplies a specific amount of food at specific times of the day and gives the owner more control over the amount eaten.

> Proprietary pet foods did not become readily available until the middle of the twentieth century.

There is a third method that is encouraged by a great many dogs and some cats, who manipulate their hapless owners with the aid of huge sorrowful eyes. It is 'feeding on demand' and needs no explanation. It should not be encouraged. Given a complete, balanced diet the pet has no need for treats or titbits and the attention it seeks can be provided (in theory) by a pat, a cuddle or by a short time spent playing with a toy.

More!

Traditionally most adult dogs are fed only once daily, even though twice daily is better for several reasons:

- the animal is less hungry after 12 hours than 24 hours and so is less likely to gorge itself
- a second meal adds interest to the day and reduces boredom; dogs who are left alone during the day are more likely to sleep after a meal
- having two meals usually reduces the amount of titbits fed; an owner will often share the breakfast toast but will be less tempted to do so if the dog has its own food
- two small meals are easier on the digestive system than one large one.

The daily ration can be divided into two equal portions or into a third and two-thirds portions.

The very large breeds of dogs appear to have relatively limited digestive capacity and so should ideally be provided with a highly digestible food. The daily amount should always be divided into two or more meals to avoid overdistension of the stomach and to ensure correct digestion.

As animals age their appetite often decreases and their digestive system is less able to cope with large amounts of food. They should be fed a minimum of two meals daily and with increasing age the daily ration should, whenever possible, be split into smaller portions so that they receive three or four small meals throughout the day.

Cats, as shown earlier, are mainly snack feeders and if possible should have food available at all times. If this is not possible, or when greedy cats are involved, food should be provided in two or more mealtimes.

TIMING OF MEALS

As always there are differing views on when animals should be fed.

'A good stockman puts his animals first' encourages owners to feed their animals before themselves. Conflicting advice says that by doing so we encourage dogs, in particular, to think they are the leader of the pack (i.e. household) and that this encourages dominance.

The good stockman feeds his animals and then goes elsewhere to feed himself. Translated to the household pet, the dog or cat is fed and then shut away from the human members of the family while they enjoy their meal. This has much to recommend it, not least because it prevents begging at the table.

However and whenever the animals are fed, the most important detail is the establishment of a routine that suits the owner and then sticking to it.

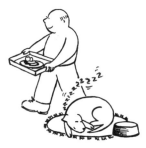

The good stockman

FEEDING SICK OR INJURED DOGS AND CATS

A food, however well formulated, is useless until eaten. Palatability plays a part but the animal must also want to eat. Sick, injured and post-op. animals need energy and nutrients to repair their damaged tissues and this should preferably be provided by the enteral route. Voluntary feeding should be encouraged whenever possible; assisted feeding is sometimes necessary but is usually a more stressful alternative.

Sick and injured animals are 'prey animals', even those of normally predator species. Their instinct is to hide away, sit tight and 'say nowt', thus drawing the minimum of attention to themselves. The strange environment of a veterinary surgery with unusual smells and noises compounds their vulnerability. Hospital cages provide few places to hide and we leave lights on for long periods or even 24 hours, thus creating unnatural and, from the animal's point of view, undesirable light patterns. The appearance of a strange two-legged animal pushing odd-smelling bowls full of dubious mix into that cage is viewed with, at best, suspicion. The surprise is that so many *do* eat.

There are many ways of persuading the reluctant eater to feed, but first of all the hydration status of the animal should be checked. Dehydration alone can cause lack of appetite, and correction of this may be sufficient for normal appetite to return. If not, try some of the following tricks which I have been taught by many animals over the years; hopefully you will not need to employ them all every time:

- Feed little and often – small amounts may whet the appetite, while large quantities will kill what little appetite exists. Little and often is also less wasteful.

Clinical tip

Check hydration status of animal before trying to feed.

- Use high-quality, energy-dense food – it is more palatable and packs in more calories per spoonful.
- Use animal-based products for both cats and dogs – sick and injured dogs utilize these better than vegetable-based ones; cats are obligate carnivores.
- Use food that is appropriate in size and texture – puppies and kittens have small mouths, small birds have small beaks.
- Mash and purée the food – 'slurp and swallow' requires less effort than 'bite and chew'.
- Feed at appropriate times – follow the home routine if possible. Crepuscular animals (e.g. rabbits) feed at dawn and dusk, nocturnal animals feed at night.
- Feed in appropriate places – arboreal animals should be fed off the ground.
- Use 'smelly' foods – appetite is stimulated by smell.
- Warm food to body temperature – create that 'fresh-killed' aroma.
- Use pottery or china dishes – some plastics absorb taints and animals often dislike the smell of metal. Remember that their nose is much more sensitive than yours.
- Use wide, flat saucers or plates – wary cats can watch for approaching danger while eating and whiskers will not touch the sides. Weak and recumbent animals can lap from plates without having to lift their heads.
- Provide suitable containers for other species – birds with damaged beaks may be unable to eat off a hard surface. They will peck seed from a full hopper as this provides 'give'. If using medicated seed in small quantities, place padding such as covered foam beneath the seed to create a softer surface.
- Accessibility – older animals or those with spinal damage may find it difficult to bend their heads to ground level, animals with splinted front leg(s) will be unable to. Immobile animals cannot move across a kennel to food placed out of reach.
- Do not place food or water next to litter trays – clean the litter tray as often as necessary and keep the cage clean to promote a pleasant environment.
- Keep the animal clean and well groomed if possible – a comfortable animal is more likely to eat.
- Ask the owner to bring the animal's own blankets and bedding – this will help the pet feel more secure.
- Use facial pheromones in the kennel to increase a cat's feeling of security.
- Provide privacy – movement draws attention to the sick animal and they will often only move to eat when they feel alone.
- Hand feed those animals that do not feel threatened by humans.

- Curiosity – try sitting by an open kennel with a cup of tea and eating biscuits while apparently ignoring the dog. 'Stray' crumbs will often disappear into the dog. This method works well on parrots too.
- Treats from home – special treats may tempt the appetite.

The last two may not provide ideal recovery foods but the first few feeds are the most important and when other methods fail anything is better than nothing. Appetite often increases once the gut has been kick-started.

- Owner visits – enlist the help of the owner. Owners who can visit and will spend time talking to, stroking and hand feeding their pet, will often succeed in persuading the animal to eat. The downside is that some owners will find very ill or badly injured animals distressing and some animals may be upset when the owner leaves. Each case must be judged on its own merits.

FORCED OR ARTIFICIAL FEEDING

If all this fails to persuade the animal to eat of its own accord or when injury prevents normal feeding, forced or artificial feeding should be instigated in order to prevent the animal becoming nutritionally compromised. Although the sick or injured animal may appear to be resting quietly, a great deal of activity is taking place within its body and lack of nutrients will impair the body's response to infection and delays healing.

In its simplest form, forced feeding involves squirting small amounts of liquid food through a syringe into the animal's mouth. The head should be held in a normal position, not raised, to reduce the high risk of aspiration pneumonia associated with this method.

The success of syringe feeding depends on the animal's ability or willingness to swallow and frequently results in more food outside the animal than in.

The tube feeding routes are more successful. The one most commonly used is the nasoenteral route, either naso-oesophageal or nasogastric tubes. The former, which ends in the oesophagus, is preferred, as the risk of gastric reflux leading to oesophagitis is considerably reduced. Naso-oesophageal tubes are easily placed, do not require anaesthetic and are well tolerated but, are of necessity, small bore tubes. They are mainly for short-term use (less than one week) though longer periods are possible. The diet used

> **Clinical tip**
>
> When force feeding, hold head in normal position to reduce risk of aspiration pneumonia.

should be balanced and easily digested. It should be free from lumps and of a 'runny' consistency; liquid enteral diets are most appropriate. In all cases of tube feeding, attention should be paid to the animal's fluid needs as well as other nutrient needs.

Placing a naso-oesophageal tube

The tube should first be measured from the nares to the seventh intercostal space in a dog or ninth rib in a cat, to ensure placement in the distal oesophagus. The length should be marked (tape is easier to see than biro markings).

The nostrils are anaesthetized with a few drops of local anaesthetic and the tip of the tube lubricated with a water-soluble lubricant. The head is held in the normal position and the tube passed into the nasal chamber and advanced into the pharynx. This should produce a swallowing reflex which allows the tube to pass into the oesophagus.

When in position, the tube should be secured as close to the nostril as possible and between and slightly above the eyes (it is better tolerated if the animal cannot see it), and an Elizabethan collar should be fitted to prevent it being dislodged.

The tube should be flushed with sterile water before use to check that it is positioned correctly. Water in the lungs will produce a cough in dogs but not always in a cat, so extra care needs to be taken when tube feeding cats. It is also possible to inject between 5 and 10 ml of air and then ausculate the stomach for borborygmi.

Flushing should also take place after use to reduce the chances of the tube blocking. If it does block, a small amount of cranberry juice will often dissolve the obstruction, but it may be better to remove the tube and start again with a new one.

Pharyngostomy tubes utilize larger bore tubes, are well tolerated and may be left in place for longer periods, but anaesthesia is required for placement. Gastrostomy tubes, for long-term use when there are oesophageal problems, also utilize larger bore tubes. They may be placed surgically or non-surgically with the aid of an endoscope, which is quicker and less traumatic. This is known as percutaneous endoscopic gastrostomy (PEG).

If it is inappropriate to use tubes which end in the oesophagus or stomach, it is possible to feed direct into the duodenum or jejunum. This requires a very small tube and the animal has to be immobilized as much as possible to reduce the risk of tube displacement. Use and management of all these tubes are covered in other texts.

Clinical tip

A small amount of cranberry juice will often dissolve an obstruction in the naso-oesophageal tube.

PARENTERAL FEEDING

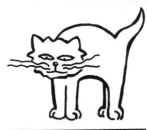

Parenteral feeding is only used when an animal cannot be fed enterally, e.g. when there is inadequate digestive or absorptive capacity, intestinal obstruction or where there is need for complete bowel rest as in acute pancreatitis or hepatitis.

By definition, parenteral feeding is the provision of adequate nutrients by intravenous injection, to maintain the animal over a relatively long period. It is expensive and time consuming. A large vein (e.g. the jugular) is required and the catheter must be placed surgically. The feeding solution is largely composed of amino acids and glucose and is an excellent growing medium for microbes so surgical standards of sterility are required for every operation.

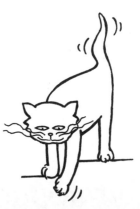

NB!

Surgical standards of sterility are required for every operation.

Definition

Parenteral feeding is the provision of adequate nutrients by intravenous injection.

Questions

1. The 'roly-poly' pup is the ideal puppy shape. True or false?
2. Which feeding method should be strongly discouraged?
3. In youth and old age, food should be offered on the little and often basis. True or false?
4. Sick and injured animals should be fed by the _____ route whenever possible.
5. When and why is artificial feeding necessary?
6. What is parenteral feeding?

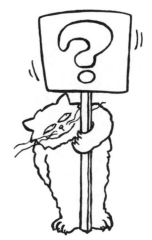

Lifestage foods

INTRODUCTION

Initially commercial foods were 'Dog' foods or 'Cat' foods. Research has refined the instinctive knowledge that animals have different nutritional requirements when they are young to when they are mature or older. Increasing levels of owner knowledge and demand has led to the production of foods that cater for the various lifestages of the dog and cat and these are now widely available from a number of manufacturers.

The research is ongoing and inevitably this will alter our present knowledge and perceptions and diets will need to be amended accordingly, so it is incumbent on all veterinary nurses to keep abreast of developments.

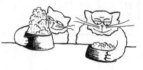

Shakespeare gave man seven ages, dogs and cats have to make do with three (or at most four) stages. These are youth (or growth), adult (maturity) and geriatric (post-maturity). The growth phase can be divided into youth and adolescence; this is particularly the case with large and giant breed dogs who have an initial rapid growth phase in common with smaller breeds, but then have a longer, slower period of growth before reaching maturity at a later age than small to medium breeds (Figure 5.1).

Nutritional requirements change in each life stage and correct nutrition will produce a healthier, happier and longer-lived pet. The life expectancy of dogs and cats has increased over the years and while many factors are involved, improved nutrition plays a significant part, helping animals to achieve their genetic potential in size as well as life expectancy. Animals in the wild rarely have a complete diet available all of the time and have evolved to be able to cope with temporary shortages of some nutrients. Although no pet diet, whether home-made or commercially prepared, can provide the ideal diet for every animal every day of its life, mainly because no one can accurately predict all the challenges that that

> It is essential that all veterinary nurses keep up with the latest developments in nutrition as research is ongoing.

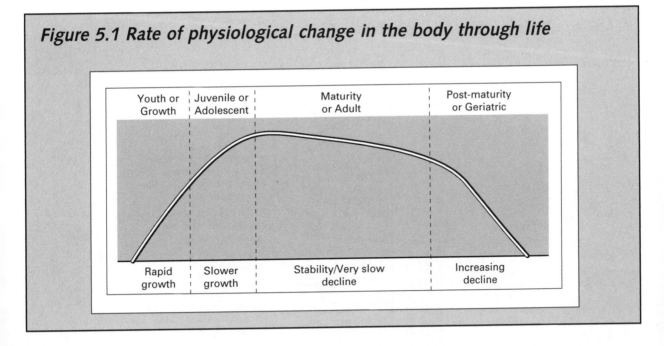

Figure 5.1 Rate of physiological change in the body through life

Youth or Growth | Juvenile or Adolescent | Maturity or Adult | Post-maturity or Geriatric

Rapid growth | Slower growth | Stability/Very slow decline | Increasing decline

animal will face, nor allow for every individual quirk of nature, a diet based on the average requirements of a group of animals at set stages of their lives, will be an improvement on nature's pot luck. Life expectancy for men and women in the developed world has increased through better provision of shelter, health-care and above all, food. The same implications are there for animals – provide a better diet and the body will operate more efficiently and last longer.

GROWTH PHASE

The growth phase starts at birth, but the neonate is a special case and will be dealt with later, so effectively the growth phase extends from weaning to that point where growth ceases.

During the growth phase the young animal has a higher requirement for protein, energy and calcium than an adult. The diet should also be high quality and easily digested. The maintenance energy requirements for puppies and kittens were given in Table 2.4. Overfeeding during the growth period should be avoided as this predisposes to skeletal problems in large dogs and obesity in all animals. The calcium to phosphorus ratio is important for correct bone and teeth formation (Figure 5.2); the optimal ratio is between 1:1 and 1.5:1.

> Overfeeding during the growth period should be avoided as this predisposes to skeletal problems in large dogs and obesity in all animals.

> The optimal ratio of calcium to phosphorus for good bone and teeth formation is 1:1–1.5:1.

Figure 5.2 Calcium and phosphorus homeostasis

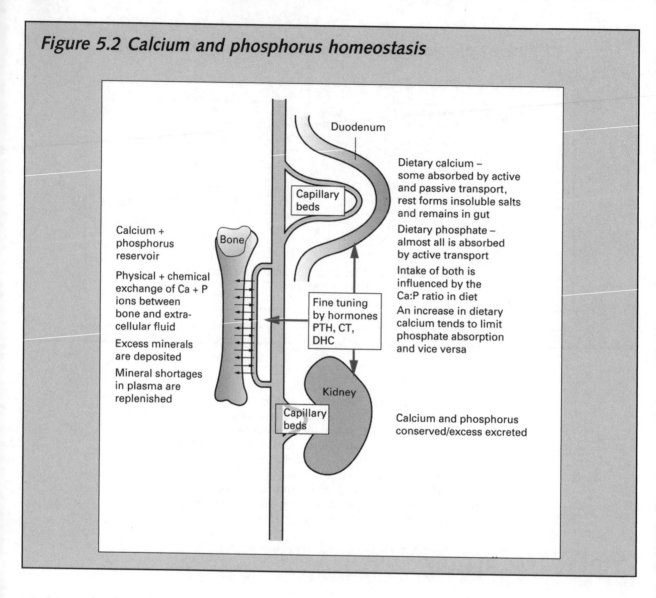

Duodenum

Capillary beds

Dietary calcium –
some absorbed by active
and passive transport,
rest forms insoluble salts
and remains in gut

Dietary phosphate –
almost all is absorbed
by active transport

Intake of both is
influenced by the
Ca:P ratio in diet

An increase in dietary
calcium tends to limit
phosphate absorption
and vice versa

Calcium + phosphorus reservoir

Physical + chemical exchange of Ca + P ions between bone and extra-cellular fluid

Excess minerals are deposited

Mineral shortages in plasma are replenished

Bone

Fine tuning
by hormones
PTH, CT,
DHC

Kidney

Capillary beds

Calcium and phosphorus
conserved/excess excreted

Severe underfeeding will prevent the animal from reaching its full adult size but slight underfeeding, while not affecting the full growth potential, appears to increase the animal's life span. This fact seems to argue against the provision of high-protein, calorie-dense foods for puppies and kittens, but it must be remembered that they have very small stomachs which limits the amount of food they can eat at any one time. If the food is of poor quality or low in energy, the young animal is unable to eat enough to satisfy its nutritional requirements. This leads to poor muscle and skeletal development, poor growth and reduced immunity. It is good practice to weigh puppies and kittens regularly to check that their growth is adequate but not excessive. Regular weighing will give a much more accurate assessment of the efficiency of the diet than appraisal by eye. Kittens should gain between 50 and 100 g per week, while puppies should gain between 2 and 4 g per day per kilogram of expected adult weight during their first 5 months. Most pups in the small and medium breed groups will reach 50% of their adult weight by the age of 4 months. Too slow a weight gain requires either extra food or a better quality one, while too rapid a weight gain suggests the use of a less energy-dense food. Roly-poly pups may look attractive but it is not an ideal start in life for them.

Establishing growth rates and nutrition levels for pups is complicated by the size range of adults. Dogs have the widest range of any species from toy to giant breeds and, because of this, the nutrient requirements will vary according to the group in which they belong. Mixed breed pups pose a particular challenge as often background information is scanty and estimating their adult size is not always easy.

Rapid growth is a major factor in the development of juvenile bone and joint disease and energy levels have the greatest impact on growth rates. In larger breeds (i.e. those whose adult weight is 25 kg or over) the aim is to feed a diet which slows down the pup's growth rate, but still enables it to reach its genetic potential at maturity. In order to do this, some restriction on the intake of nutrients is needed. This can be achieved by changing to an 'adolescent' diet in which the protein and energy levels fall between those of 'growth' foods and 'adult' foods, at around 5 months, or by restricting intake – feeding a fixed amount twice daily. Modified growth foods for large breeds are now available with energy levels adjusted to prevent these breeds from growing too quickly. These produce a more even growth curve than a combination of high-energy growth and slightly reduced energy adolescent foods. (This development is an illustration of dietary knowledge being modified by further research.) Regular weighing will again provide a check on progress and adjustments can be made accordingly.

ADULT PHASE

The adult stage is that time after the animal ceases to grow and before visual and physiological changes due to the ageing process begin to appear. Smaller breeds of dogs mature earlier than large ones and age slower,

The adult stage is that time after the animal ceases to grow and before visual and physiological changes due to the ageing process begin to appear.

so that for small breeds the adult phase will be a significant part of their lives. Large and giant breeds mature later and age quickly, so the adult phase is comparatively short in these dogs. In cats the adult phase is usually reckoned to last from about one year to around 7 years of age, similar to small dogs.

For the majority of animals, with the exception of working dogs, toy breeds and pregnant or lactating animals, nutritional needs in this phase are the least demanding and are met by any good-quality pet food. A check should always be kept on weight and body condition score, although this can be done less frequently than during the growth phase. The amount fed should always be linked to the amount of exercise the animal receives and it is important to remember that feeding advice on the tin or packet are only recommendations, not absolute quantities. The weight and body condition score will indicate whether the amount being fed is correct or requires adjustment. The aim is to maintain the animal's ideal body weight by balancing the amount fed with the activity levels so that the animal enters its post-maturity phase as healthy as possible.

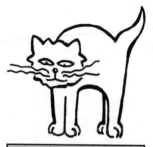

NB!
Feeding instructions included on pet food labels are for guidance only and not absolute quantities.

Working dogs

These dogs will have a higher than normal energy requirement and those who work outside in adverse weather conditions will have even higher energy demands. In many cases increasing the amount of food offered is not sufficient; an energy-dense food ensures the animal can eat enough to satisfy its energy requirements. Stomach capacity is limited and working dogs at the end of the day may be too tired to eat large quantities of low-energy food.

Dogs whose energy needs vary at different times of the year should be fed normal adult rations during their non-working periods. A gradual changeover to the more calorie-dense food should start 1–2 weeks prior to need to allow the body to adjust its digestive mechanisms.

Toy dogs

Toy breeds, which often have very small appetites and small stomach capacity, may also benefit from being fed a calorie-dense food but a careful watch should be kept on their weight and body condition score.

The extra energy for both working and toy dogs is best supplied in the form of fat, first because fat contains more calories per unit weight than protein or carbohydrate, and secondly because dogs appear to utilize the energy stored in fat more efficiently. The use of fat for energy also avoids the necessity to remove from the body the waste products that occur when protein is used.

PREGNANCY AND LACTATION

While the production of offspring is essential for continuation of the species, nature regards the reproductive system as a non-essential system. This seemingly contradictory statement actually makes sense because, in a time of food shortages, pups and kittens will be born, at best, weak and without the supply of nourishment that a healthy dam would be able to produce. The likelihood is that they would not survive to maturity – in nature's view a waste of energy and nutrients. Consequently, in times of shortage, nutrients are directed first to the essential organs, heart, brain, kidneys, etc., in the hope that the animal will survive long enough for better times to arrive.

Such an extreme is unlikely to occur in companion animals but it does emphasize the need for optimal health in those animals intended for breeding. The production of a healthy and vigorous litter should be the aim of breeders and efforts are usually concentrated on the dam, but the role of the sire should not be overlooked. It is important that he is in optimal health to ensure adequate production of healthy sperm. In both sexes optimal reproductive efficiency depends on many factors, including adequate energy concentrations, adequate supplies of essential fatty acids and a balanced supply of vitamins and minerals, both at the time of conception and prior to it. Animals intended for breeding should be fed a good-quality balanced diet designed for adult maintenance.

Pregnancy, as women are frequently told, is not an illness, it is a natural condition but one that places extra demands and constraints on the body. This is no less true for animals.

The fetus requires adequate nutrition for correct growth and development and it is of course the dam that supplies this. It is therefore, reasonable to assume that nutritional inadequacies in the dam will be reflected in the development of the fetus. Ideally the bitch or queen will end lactation weighing the same as at the start of the pregnancy, but to do so the increased nutrient and energy demands require her to have an

> Nature regards the reproductive system as a non-essential system.

increased intake of both during pregnancy and lactation.

There are two ways of providing this added requirement during pregnancy:

- a larger quantity of the usual diet
- a more concentrated diet provided in the same or slightly increased quantity than the normal diet.

Lactation places even greater demands on her body and a concentrated diet is the best way to provide the extra energy, protein and other nutrients.

Bitches

The bitch does not have a large increase in tissue growth in the first half of pregnancy and for the first 4–5 weeks a normal amount of the usual diet should suffice, provided that it is a good-quality balanced food. At this point the amount fed can start to be gradually increased so that at whelping she is receiving around 50% more than her normal quantity. Alternatively, during the fifth week a puppy food can be slowly introduced to replace her usual food. After the fifth week the amount fed can be slightly increased so that by the time of whelping she will be consuming up to 20% extra. Her weight at this time should be approximately 20% greater than at the start of pregnancy but this will depend to some extent on the size of the litter.

In the last 2 weeks the pups will take up more and more space in her abdomen, so the bitch's stomach capacity is severely limited, particularly if she is carrying a large litter. Small, frequent meals are required at this stage.

Lactation places enormous strains on the bitch's resources. The peak demand from the pups comes 3 weeks after birth. At this stage the bitch's energy needs can be three to four times her own MER. The requirements for other nutrients are similarly high and an energy-dense, high-quality protein, highly digestible food should be provided ad lib.

Lactating bitches also require large quantities of fluid, so fresh drinking water should always be available. Many owners feel that lactating bitches (and queens) require milk in order to produce milk, but unfortunately this is not as logical as it sounds. Many animals are not able to digest lactose (milk sugar) and some are sensitive to milk proteins. These animals will have to cope with extra stress on the digestive system when large amounts of milk are offered, stress that is best avoided.

Queens

The pregnant queen, unlike the bitch, has an increased need for energy and nutrients from the start of her pregnancy. The extra nutrients may again be supplied by increasing the amount of her normal diet or by changing to a more concentrated diet. When fed her normal diet she will regulate her appetite to ensure the required increases are met, but providing a more energy-dense diet will enable her to meet requirements with the same quantity of food. When stomach capacity is limited in the later stages of pregnancy this is of obvious benefit to the queen.

Lactation again places high demands on the mother and a highly digestible, good-quality protein, energy-dense food should be fed at this time. This can be offered ad lib or as small, frequent meals. Fluid intake is important and fresh water should always be available

When the puppies and kittens are weaned, the stimulating effect of suckling will be removed and the mother's food and fluid intake should be reduced to discourage the further production of milk. The bitch or queen should be gradually changed back to a maintenance diet, although if they have lost a lot of weight and condition, keeping them on an energy-dense diet for a short while will be beneficial. The bitch or queen should be back to normal amounts of her normal diet within 3–4 weeks of the puppies or kittens being weaned.

NEONATES

As most neonates will be fed and tended by their mothers, it is appropriate to include them here.

The optimal diet for the neonate is its own mother's milk. Not only will it be nutritionally balanced for that particular species, but it will also provide antibodies and other proteins, which encourage the correct development of the immature gut. Hormones, enzymes and growth factors are also present and these play an important role in the health and development of the animal.

Hand-reared pups and kittens tend to do less well than maternally reared animals, partly because replacement milks are not able to provide all the extras, but ensuring that they receive some of the first milk (colostrum) will help mitigate these deficiencies.

The concentrations of several nutrients present in the milk of bitches and queens change through

Fact

The milk of bitches and queens changes in composition throughout lactation to meet the changing needs of their offspring.

lactation to meet the changing needs of their offspring. As an example, the energy content of the milk increases during the first 5 weeks to meet the increasing energy needs of the puppies or kittens. Milk replacer does not do this and extra energy requirements have to be met by extra volume, which is not always adequate or satisfactory.

Commonly pups and kittens will start to eat semi-solid food soon after the eruption of the temporary teeth, but milk remains sufficient to sustain growth and development up to 4–5 weeks of age. The nutritional quality of the milk is maintained at the expense of the bitch or queen's own body if necessary, but when their diet is very poor or quantities are insufficient, the milk supply may fail and the pups or kittens will need extra nutritional support.

Weaning should be a gradual process to allow time for the immature gut to adapt to differently sourced nutrients and should be matched to the capability of the individual to tolerate solid food. It is important to bear in mind that these immature digestive systems function best with meat protein and animal fats. Cereal is not really appropriate at this stage, although traditionally it has been fed to pups. When the dam is fed a growth food during lactation, it is likely that the puppies and kittens will start to eat this and are thus weaned onto an appropriate food with the minimum of fuss.

After weaning, milk is not essential and with the animal's declining ability to digest lactose, the possibility of dietary intolerance to milk increases.

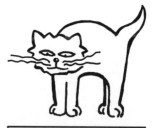

NB!
Immature digestive systems function best with meat protein and animal fats.

GERIATRIC STAGE

The geriatric or post-maturity stage follows on from the maturity phase and continues until death. In small breeds of dogs this phase begins around 7 or 8 years of age, at 5 years in large and giant breeds and 7 years in the cat. In many animals this will equate to a third or more of its life span. Certain breeds such as the Border Collie and Jack Russell, which are known for their longevity, probably have a later onset for the post-maturity phase, but little research appears to have been done in this field.

Since by definition maturity ends before visual and physiological changes appear, the tissues, organs and systems of the animal must deteriorate through the post-maturity phase, becoming gradually less efficient and eventually failing. Although this is a natural process, its progression can be managed and acceptable levels of activity and well-being maintained for a reasonable period.

Onset of old age:

Small dog breeds ± 7/8 years
Large dog breeds ± 5 years
Cat ± 7 years

The rate of deterioration is dependent on several factors, including environment and genetic make-up, but nutrition and nutritional history are major factors. An animal at its optimal weight and having received a good diet throughout its life will enter the post-maturity phase with the prospect of several healthy years still to come.

Changes noticed by the owner may include greying, particularly of the muzzle, and a general slowing down and stiffness after rest. However, these changes are usually very gradual and because of this may not be noticed for some time. They may also notice changes in eating habits and the quantity of water drunk. Many owners accept these changes, simply putting them down to 'getting older' and do little about them until they become a severe nuisance, e.g. excessive drinking in a dog leading to excessive urination. Although this may be noticed earlier, the owner will often not mention it until the dog can no longer last through the night. At this point the owner is faced with either morning puddles or a broken night's sleep when their pet demands to be let out in the early hours, and begins to wonder 'if something can be done'. Polydipsia and polyuria can be symptoms of several conditions, including diabetes mellitus and kidney disease, treatment for both of which will include dietary modification to help manage and slow progression of the disease. The earlier the condition is noticed and diagnosed, the more effective the dietary modification will be, so owners should be encouraged to report such signs early.

To be fully effective, dietary modification should commence before or as soon as ageing signs become detectable. Formulating a diet for older animals needs to take into consideration the changes taking place in the animal's body, which will affect the energy requirements and the relative amounts of nutrients that should be supplied. Body composition changes with age and alters the requirement for energy as we have seen earlier. Weight for weight, body fat stores need less energy than muscle mass. Body fat stores increase until middle age and then tend to decrease, but lean body mass (skeletal muscle) tends to reduce with age, altering the ratio of muscle to body fat. (This reduction in lean body mass is part of the natural ageing process but also occurs throughout life when the body enters negative nitrogen balance, i.e. when protein degradation exceeds synthesis.)

Skeletal muscle is lost in preference to muscle tissue from the heart, liver and digestive tract. Loss of skeletal muscle not only leads to reduced physical activity, it effectively reduces the reserves of amino acids available for tissue repair and energy metabolism and so is likely to reduce the body's ability to respond to physical trauma, stress and infections. It is in the animal's best interest to maintain this muscle mass for as long as possible and to this end it is important to encourage exercise in older animals as the body maintains muscle that is used.

Impaired kidney function is a major concern in older animals and it is often recommended that protein levels are reduced in diets for these animals, but there are conflicting views on the value of doing so. Some claim that restricting protein protects the kidneys, while others maintain that protein reduction is not necessary until clinical signs of kidney failure appear. Given that a large part of kidney function is lost by this stage, it makes sense to mildly restrict protein prior to clinical signs appearing. Protein levels should not, however, be reduced to a level that fails to support the skeletal muscle mass. Perhaps of more concern is protein quality, high-quality protein supplying the necessary amounts of amino acids with minimal waste to be disposed of. Restriction of dietary phosphorus is, however, recommended to protect and support ageing kidneys and liver.

Kidney function deterioration may lead to increased loss of water-soluble vitamins and an increased dietary supply is recommended to compensate. Impaired kidney function, linked to a reduced sensitivity to thirst, may lead to dehydration, so particular attention should be paid to the animal's fluid intake, particularly those fed a dry food. For this reason and others, including loss of jaw muscle tone and dental problems, changing to a tinned or other moist diet (more palatable and easier to eat) will often improve the older animal's intake of fluids and nutrients with a consequent improvement in health and condition.

Immunocompetence, or resistance to infection, another concern in older animals, is affected by protein levels because antibodies are formed from proteins, but antioxidant levels are also important. Impaired digestive function can lead to the production of extra free radicals, while the impaired uptake of vitamins and minerals may lead to reduced antioxidant levels. Increasing the levels of antioxidants in the diet is usually considered to be beneficial, particularly vitamin E which is indicated in cardiovascular protection. Although some elderly animals are overweight, it is important that their diet contains a reasonable level of fat to ensure adequate uptake of fat-soluble vitamins, especially vitamin E.

The cat, as an obligate carnivore, appears to be particularly sensitive to protein restriction and in the normal healthy cat there is little reason to restrict the amount of protein fed. This applies even in old age and a level of 30% protein has been suggested for cats to maintain lean body mass.

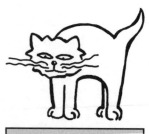

NB!
It is important to encourage exercise in older animals as the body maintains muscle that is used.

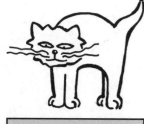

NB!
Kidney function deterioration may lead to increased loss of water-soluble vitamins and an increased dietary supply is recommended.

It is usually recommended that fat levels are reduced in diets designed for older animals to compensate for reduction in activity levels and to guard against obesity; however, some older cats, over the age of 12 years, seem to suffer from an energy deficiency which exacerbates the reduction in lean body mass and these cases require more energy rather than less. This energy is best supplied by increasing the dietary fat levels.

All animals are individuals and it is therefore difficult to generalize (even though this book attempts to do so), and it is in the geriatric phase where generalizations are least appropriate. The whole body is degenerating, but different systems do so at different rates, so that one animal may show reduced kidney function while another may have satisfactory renal function but have impaired liver function. Yet another may appear normal, but a period of stress will reveal that functional reserves in one or more systems have been severely impaired. The combinations and computations are seemingly endless, so it is particularly important in this phase to tailor the diet to the individual and to be prepared to modify it as and when necessary.

> It is particularly important in the geriatric phase to tailor the diet to the individual patient.

Questions

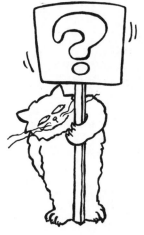

1. What is the optimal calcium to phosphorus ratio in the diet for correct bone and teeth formation in dogs and cats?
2. The level of energy in the diet is the most important controller of growth rates. True or false?
3. The amount of food fed to an adult dog should be in proportion to the amount of exercise it receives. True or false?
4. Energy-dense diets should only be fed to working dogs. True or false?
5. List three reasons why its mother's milk is the best food for the neonate.
6. Milk is sufficient to sustain growth and development for up to _____ __ _____ weeks.
7. Animals should continue to receive milk as an essential part of their diet throughout life. True or false?
8. Encouraging _____ maintains _____ muscle mass.

6

The gut as an ecosystem

INTRODUCTION

Unfortunately not all animals remain healthy throughout their lives. Accident, disease or organ malfunction can all cause problems and often surgical or medical intervention will be necessary. In almost all cases, modification of the diet will assist recovery, slow the progression of incurable disease or ameliorate the effects of organ dysfunction.

In some cases, adjustment of the quantities and proportions of nutrients is sufficient to improve the animal's health, in others a more complex manipulation is required when we need to consider not just a particular nutrient but a particular type of that nutrient and its effect on the whole body. To understand this we need to take an overall view and realize that the digestive tract is not just a conveyor belt through the body, but a complete ecosystem.

By definition an ecosystem has two components, a community of organisms (the biotic component) and their habitat. The organisms interact with each other, often competing for space and food, and are influenced by the chemical and physical features of their environment (the abiotic component). The biotic component in the gut is formed of bacteria, fungi, protozoa, yeasts and other organisms. Their numbers vary in different sections of the digestive tract, tending to increase in numbers distally. The acidity of the stomach prevents high numbers there and rapid transit of food through the upper regions of the bowel normally discourages proliferation of organisms but, in the large intestine, and in particular the colon, high numbers of microorganisms flourish. They are able to do so because the food residues are present in greater quantity and the flow rate is slower; their effect on the body of the host animal is therefore greatest in the colon.

The composition of the gut flora is established within 2–3 weeks of birth through contact with the mother and her environment. Once organisms colo-

> The composition of the gut flora is established within 2–3 weeks of birth.

nize the gut, they are generally there for life, but their relative proportions can be influenced by the diet of the animal. Most of the research into the biotic component of the gastrointestinal ecosystem has concerned bacteria, the function and importance of the other microorganisms being, as yet, not fully understood.

Gut bacteria fall into three groups – the good, the bad and the indifferent – or to put it more scientifically, the beneficial species (bifidobacteria and eubacteria together with lactobacilli and other lactic acid bacteria), the pathogenic and putrefactive species (enterobacteria and clostridia) and neutral species (effectively the rest). These bacteria are part of the ecosystem, interacting with each other and the environment, but chiefly living their own lives and producing their own waste. This waste may be of use to the host animal, e.g. short-chain fatty acids which are used as a source of energy by the cells lining the colon, or may damage the host, e.g. toxic or carcinogenic products. If the beneficial bacteria can be increased in numbers, then the beneficial effects on the host will be greater. Greater numbers of these will also tend to crowd out the pathogens (this is known as exclusion by competition) and so reduce the harmful effects. It is also possible that the beneficial bacteria may produce substances toxic to the pathogens and that beneficial bacteria boost the body's ability to resist the potential toxic effects of pathogens.

It is possible to manipulate these bacterial populations in two ways:

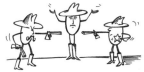

The good, the bad and the indifferent

- provide beneficial bacteria as a dietary supplement – probiotics
- provide substrates to encourage increase of beneficial bacteria – prebiotics.

PROBIOTICS

Probiotics are live, natural products given by mouth in the hope that they will colonize the gut and so improve the balance of the resident microorganisms, restoring or maintaining normal gut function. Their use is indicated in a wide range of situations, e.g. in times of stress and in old age, but perhaps the strongest indication for their use is when the normal gut bacteria levels are severely damaged. Antibacterial therapy, heavy parasite burdens causing gut damage and gut infections all have the effect of depressing

> Probiotics are live, natural products given by mouth, e.g. Brewer's yeast and yoghurt.

bacterial populations and may create conditions which favour the growth of pathogens. Use of probiotics at these times will replace the lost beneficial bacteria.

There are a number of products available; some supplements consist of bacteria alone, others include yeasts, for example Brewer's yeast, which has traditionally been used as a supplement for dogs and cats and is a good source of thiamin. It is often recommended that dogs are given yoghurt as an aid to recovery from gastrointestinal upsets. This contains beneficial *Lactobacillus* species, but it needs to be a live culture to be effective.

In many cases, the addition of live yoghurt or other probiotics to the diet does appear to have a beneficial influence on the gut bacteria populations despite the fact that the validity of the exercise has been questioned by those who doubt the ability of the organisms to survive in the acidic environment of the stomach. However, gastrointestinal upsets caused by the ingestion of contaminated material would seem to imply that if the contamination is sufficiently high, some microorganisms will survive the acid onslaught in the stomach and pass through to the intestines to cause problems there. If this is the case, then provided that the food is seeded with a high number of live beneficial bacteria, sufficient will pass through to colonize the small and large intestines.

PREBIOTICS

The use of prebiotics relies on the adaptability of organisms. Population size (i.e. how many there are of any one type of organism) depends on several factors, including the total amount of food available and the competition from other species. If one organism can adapt itself to take advantage of a situation that other species cannot, then it will thrive while other species decrease. This is termed adaptability. In the case of the gut flora, a feature common to the beneficial bacteria is their ability to ferment fibre. Pathogens and putrefying bacteria seem less able to do this, so the presence of fermentable fibre will encourage an increase in beneficial bacteria and a corresponding decrease in pathogens. Conversely, a poor diet tends to favour the increase of pathogenic bacteria. Prebiotics are substances that are able to alter the gut flora in favour of the beneficial microorganisms. Fermentable fibres and in particular the fructo-oligosaccharides, are the most effective prebiotics in modifying favourable gut populations and metabolic effects in the gastro-intestinal tract.

The effects of probiotics on the gut flora may only be temporary if beneficial populations are not able to multiply faster than the pathogens. Prebiotics lay the foundations for more permanent manipulation of the gut flora by encouraging growth and development of beneficial populations, while limiting development of pathogenic populations. For maximum effect we should perhaps consider utilizing both pre- and probiotics by using a probiotic supplement along with an adequate supply of fermentable fibre in the diet.

Manipulation of the gut flora by diet to encourage growth of beneficial populations has several results including:

- inhibition of harmful bacteria with a corresponding reduction in toxins, carcinogens and putrefactive substances
- stimulation of the immune system
- increased absorption and utilization of nutrients
- increased synthesis of vitamins
- improved stool characteristics
- increased production of the short-chain fatty acids (SCFAs), acetate, butyrate and propionic.

These SCFAs are used as metabolic substrates by body tissues and are rapidly absorbed into the epithelial cells of the colon where they are utilized or passed into the bloodstream. Butyrate is known to be an important fuel for colonocytes in some species and may also be important in dogs. Although fermentation by bacteria is most likely to occur in the colon, some fermentation does take place in the small intestine and dogs fed a diet containing fermentable fibre usually have larger and heavier than normal small intestines with a corresponding increase in mucosal and absorptive surface areas, which together have beneficial effects for the animal.

Bacterial populations in the gut require nitrogen for growth. Some of this will come from the animal's diet, but an important source of nitrogen for bacteria in the large intestine is blood urea diffusing into the bowel. It is then broken down by enzymes (ureases) and used by the bacteria for protein synthesis. This bacterial protein eventually passes out of the animal in the faeces. High populations of bacteria therefore reduce levels of blood urea and lessen the need for it to be excreted through the kidneys, so we can add a renoprotective role to the list of benefits of fermentable fibre in the diet.

FATTY ACIDS AND EICOSANOIDS

The effects of fermentable fibre on bacterial populations is one example of how different types of the same dietary component (in this case fibre) produce different effects in the body. Similarly different types of fatty acids have different effects.

Figure 6.1 Formation of saturated and unsaturated fatty acids

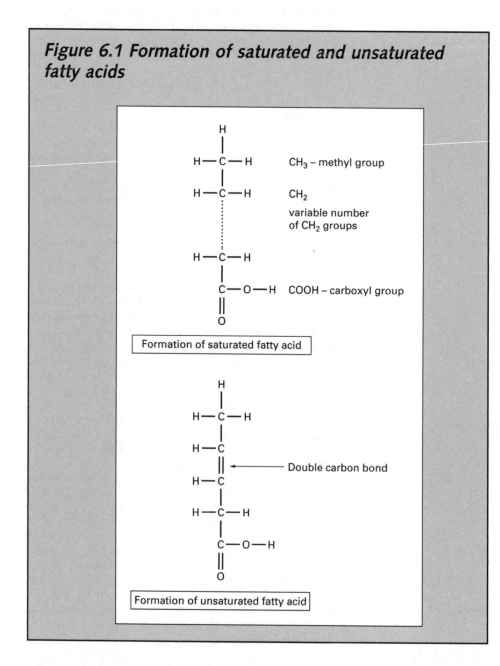

Fats and oils, as we have already seen, are lipids which occur in two forms, single or conjugated lipids. Nothing in nature is that simple though and fatty acids can be further divided into saturated and unsaturated compounds. Saturated fatty acids are linear carbon chains occurring chiefly in animals. Unsaturated fatty acids contain double bonds and occur chiefly in plants. Figure 6.1 compares the formation of saturated and unsaturated fatty acids.

Adding a double bond to the linear saturated fatty acid promotes twisting so that unsaturated fatty acids take up more space and are less tightly packed in biological membranes.

The variable number of carbon atoms in the chains leads to a wide variety of fats. Both saturated and unsaturated normally contain even numbers of carbon atoms, with proprionic acid providing an exception with three carbon atoms.

Unsaturated carbon atoms may contain one double bond (monounsaturated) or two or more double bonds (polyunsaturated). These double bonds occur at different positions along the chain, giving rise to different classes of polyunsaturated fatty acids (PUFAs). The position of the first double bond in the carbon chain (the carbon of the CH_3 group is taken as number one) names the class of PUFA. Figure 6.2 illustrates two examples of these PUFA classes.

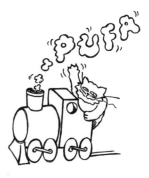

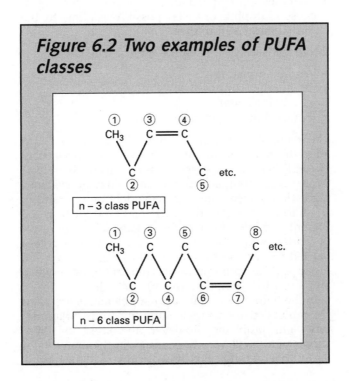

Figure 6.2 Two examples of PUFA classes

n – 3 class PUFA

n – 6 class PUFA

The essential fatty acids, linoleic and arachidonic acid, are members of the n − 6 class and naturally occurring linolenic acid belongs to the n − 3 class. Generally speaking, animals cannot convert n − 6 fatty acids to n − 3 fatty acids or vice versa (linolenic acid produced from linoleic acid is slightly different to that naturally occurring) so the amounts of n − 6 and n − 3 fatty acids in the body are dependent on those present in the diet.

Algae synthesize large amounts of n–3 fatty acids and so most marine animals have high concentrations of n − 3 fatty acids in their bodies. Plants, on the other hand, contain a higher percentage of n − 6 fatty acids so that terrestrial animals consuming these plants have a higher concentration of n − 6 fatty acids in their bodies.

Eicosanoids are compounds derived from polyunsaturated fatty acids in the cell membranes. They act as a type of hormone and are responsible for regulation of normal physiology and play a part in the body's inflammatory responses. They are not stored in the body but synthesized as required, arachidonic acid being their main precursor. However, the type synthesized is dependent on the type of fatty acid released from the cell membrane.

Eicosanoids derived from arachidonic acid (n − 6) are:

- proinflammatory
- immunosuppressive and
- cause clumping of cells (possibly leading to the formation of a thrombus).

Eicosanoids derived from n − 3 fatty acids are:

- less inflammatory
- not immunosuppressive
- vasodilatory and
- reduce clumping of cells.

The manipulation of dietary lipids has the potential to affect the animal's inflammatory responses in a variety of conditions and illnesses. However, as n − 6 and n − 3 fatty acids compete for the same enzyme systems, regulation of eicosanoids is dependent on the ratio of n − 6 to n − 3 rather than the total amount of n − 3 present. A predominance of n − 6 fatty acids will result in a proinflammatory state. The inflammatory potential reduces as the amount of n − 3 relative to n − 6 increases. The optimum ratio is thought to be between 5 (n − 6):1 (n − 3) and 10 (n − 6):1 (n − 3).

In the light of this, fatty acid supplements are often recommended for animals suffering from inflammatory skin problems, however, the effect of these supplements will vary depending on the amounts of n − 6 and n − 3 fatty acids already present in the diet.

Fatty acid supplements given with a diet containing low amounts of n – 6 fatty acids will tip the balance further towards the desirable ratio than they will when the diet contains high amounts of n – 6 fatty acids. For this reason a diet which has been designed to contain the desirable ratio of n – 6: n – 3 is likely to be more effective than supplementation, as it gives greater control over the total quantities of n – 6 and n – 3 and therefore the ratio between them, in the diet.

Questions

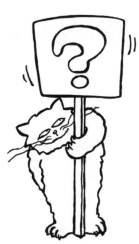

1. List three types of organism which form the biotic component of the gut's ecosystem.
2. Name two beneficial bacteria.
3. What is 'exclusion by competition'?
4. What are prebiotics?
5. What are eicosanoids?

$$\overset{\textstyle 7}{\bigcirc}$$

Clinical nutrition

INTRODUCTION

So feeding a good-quality, balanced diet, paying attention to the provision of fermentable fibre and the correct ratio of n – 6 to n – 3 PUFAs, will keep the animal on the straight and narrow path of health – well maybe, but despite our best efforts, animals do become ill.

Although a poor or incorrect diet may in some cases lead to the condition occurring, dietary changes rarely *cure* disease or disorders – they are a way of managing the problem. Providing nutritional support in any illness increases the chances of survival; dietary changes may prevent deterioration or at least slow down the progression of a disease and by avoiding nutrients that produce symptoms, the animal's quality of life can be improved.

When choosing a diet for a sick animal, it is important to think of the animal as a whole, as there may be more than one condition present that requires nutritional consideration. When this happens, the most life-threatening condition should take precedence. It is also important to take the lifestage of the animal into account; for example, a puppy with a renal condition will require a different diet to an adult or old dog with kidney disease.

Vets will often recommend and owners will often choose to feed a proprietary clinical diet for ease, convenience and consistency, but it is possible to prepare home-made diets for these various conditions, although such recipes are outside the scope of this book. (Information on home-prepared alternatives is available from some of the clinical diet manufacturers). Under certain circumstances home prepared is best. Animals suffering from clinical conditions are almost always malnourished and often inappetant or anorexic. It is important that whenever possible they eat and home-prepared diets are more acceptable to many pets at these times.

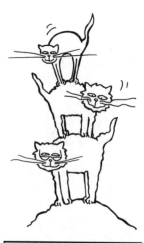

Fact

Dietary changes are a management tool – not a cure for disease.

When the gut is compromised it can become permeable to large molecules that would not normally pass through and there is a danger of hypersensitivities developing. In these circumstances it is helpful if the animal is fed products it will not normally encounter and home-made diets can be adapted to allow for this.

Ultimately, any disease and its consequences will affect the whole body, but it is customary to classify disease according to which body system it originates in.

BODY SYSTEMS

- Structural
  - skeletal
  - muscular
  - integument
  - cardiovascular
- Visceral
  - digestive
  - respiratory
  - urinary
  - reproductive
- Coordinating
  - nervous
  - endocrine

From a dietary management point of view, the muscular and nervous systems are considered together, i.e. neuromuscular. Diet has effectively little or no direct effect on the respiratory system and is therefore disregarded here.

There are two occasions when malnutrition profoundly affects the whole body, obesity and starvation in its various forms, and these are dealt with first.

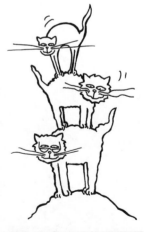

OBESITY

Obesity is easily recognized and seen frequently, while its occurrence and ill effects have been widely publicized. In humans it has spawned multimillion pound businesses dedicated to its eradication and yet the size of the problem is (literally) increasing in both humans and pets.

So much has already been written about obesity in pets that it is tempting to gloss over it here, but it is

Fact
Prevention is better than cure.

included because it is important and it is important because:

- it is the most common nutritional disease seen in practice (and in the street) in the dog, cat and increasingly in other pets
- it affects all organs and functions of the body, usually adversely
- it is preventable! There are hundreds of overweight animals, but there are hundreds more who potentially could benefit from the old maxim – *prevention is better than cure*.

Veterinary nurses should preach to their clients from day 1 of pet ownership that:

Overfeeding = Overweight = Decreased quality of life for their pet

If a veterinary nurse does nothing else, by educating clients into owning slim pets, he or she will have helped many animals to have a healthier life.

Obesity can have several causes. Occasionally there are underlying medical reasons why an animal is overweight but, almost always, obesity is due to the ingestion of too many calories linked with too low levels of physical activity. The availability of highly palatable, energy-dense diets without a corresponding recognition that less of these diets needs to be fed, only exacerbates the problem.

Genetic factors are almost certainly involved, as is implied by the tendency of certain breeds (and their crosses) to be overweight and it is true that some dogs, regardless of breed, live only to eat, with disastrous consequences to their figures. These latter cases are particularly difficult to deal with.

Leptin is a hormone that has been shown to influence appetite and metabolic rate in man and in mice. It is produced by fat cells and acts on sites within the hypothalamus, with high levels of leptin decreasing appetite and low levels stimulating it (Figure 7.1). Mice with low levels of leptin had insatiable appetites, low energy output and were obese. For a time it was thought that a cure for obesity had been found – inject the mice with leptin and all would be well, appetite would decrease and weight would be lost – and in the leptin-deficient mice (and humans) this did happen. Unfortunately, as might have been expected, the answer was not that simple. Overweight people with a leptin deficit are few on the ground; indeed because of their increased fat levels, most produce higher than average amounts of leptin. So the answer to this problem lies elsewhere. It may lie with the receptor sites or with faulty pathways or with other, as yet, unknown factors. Research is continuing but meanwhile there can be no doubt that

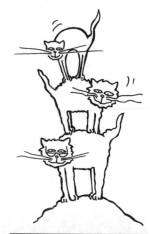

> **Fact**
> Overfeeding =
> Overweight =
> Decreased quality of life

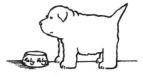

I'm just cuddly

obesity is a serious problem, and that successful treatment is a challenge, made more difficult by the fact that owner recognition and determination to treat the disease is perhaps more important than the actual diet. For every success story there are several more failures or relapses, so we come back to the importance of prevention.

The percentage of body fat increases as animals grow, from 1 to 2% at birth, through 10 to 15% at 6 months, to around 20% as an adult. This level is normal. It is also normal for females to have a higher body fat ratio than males and for the percentage of body fat to increase in older animals as the percentage of lean body mass decreases. What is not normal is excessive fat.

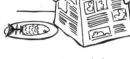

A mature cat needs less food

New fat cells are laid down during growth to accommodate the normal increase in body fat levels. Each of these cells has a basic volume, below which it will not shrink except at times of severe food shortages. If excess calories are consumed at this stage, extra fat cells will be formed and will be present for life (except again under conditions of extreme deprivation). The roly-poly pup, although cuddly and much loved by owners, has been burdened with a problem for life.

Adolescence is also a critical time when, as the animal nears maturity, its appetite often appears to decrease in response to the body's reduced need for energy and protein. This is most noticeable in pups that have been fed non-lifestage foods during growth. These foods are likely to have contained inadequate levels of energy and protein for growth and the animal has had to eat higher than normal amounts to satisfy its requirements. With the onset of maturity, the phase these foods are best suited to, food consumption will drop causing many owners to worry about this perceived lack of appetite and they will encourage their pet to eat at the previously high levels. These owners need to be reassured that, in the healthy animal, this decrease is normal. A further complication often occurring at this time is neutering. Neutering tends to decrease activity in both males and females and linked with the removal of oestrogen and testosterone, both of which have appetite depressant effects, increases the tendency of the animal to become overweight. 'Overweight' is, however, a term which should be used with care. Muscle is heavier, volume for volume, than fat and athletic or working animals with well-developed muscles, may have weights which are over the breed average, but not have excess fat stores. Body condition score should always be considered alongside weight.

Dietary management of obesity can take several forms. Dogs which receive large numbers of treats

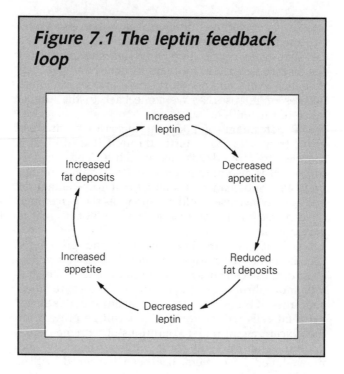

Figure 7.1 The leptin feedback loop

(often fat-laden chews) or human left-overs, without a corresponding decrease in their food ration, will benefit from the removal of these factors from their diet. On occasion this is all that is needed.

In the early stages of obesity, cutting down on the amounts of food fed or changing to a slightly less calorie dense diet may be sufficient.

In severe cases, the calorie restriction required demands the use of specially formulated diets if the supply of other essential nutrients is not to be compromised. There are several different diets of this type available, each with its own advantages and disadvantages, and different animals will lose weight better on different diets.

Weight loss programmes aim for a reduction of 15% bodyweight over a period of 3 months, and the recommended daily amounts of reduced-calorie diets are calculated with this in mind. It is usually beneficial to split this quantity into two or three small meals and exercise should be considered an integral part of the programme.

All commercially produced calorie-reduced diets contain less fat than normal maintenance diets (fat is more energy dense than carbohydrate or protein and is more efficiently digested and utilized by dogs and cats), but vary in the addition of fibre, air or moisture. Fibre is added to produce a feeling of satiety or 'fullness' in the animal, thus reducing the amount eaten. The extent to which fibre levels affect satiety is debated but increasing fibre content can slow down the digestion and absorption of nutrients, and so reduce the uptake of calories from the food. Fibre has the disadvantage of increasing the amount of faeces passed and this may not be acceptable to all owners. Air and moisture are added to maintain the volume of the food so that the quantity fed remains the same but contains fewer calories. This may be more important to the owner than the animal.

Finding the right diet can be a matter of trial and error and can take time. It is important to remember that not only must the diet be acceptable to the dog or cat, it must also be acceptable to the owner.

Weight loss should be gradual and is a long-term project. Losing weight is as much about re-educating the owner on feeding regimens, as it is about supplying a low-calorie diet. Owners need encouragement and reassurance over a long period – instant results are not on offer – but the eventual rewards are worth waiting for: a happier, healthier, more active pet that will live longer.

STARVATION

Starvation, the opposite extreme to obesity, is thankfully seen much less often. Most veterinary nurses will only rarely see the animal that is reduced to 'skin and bone'. These severely emaciated animals are extremely fragile, because not only has the body been deprived of food, the gastrointestinal tract has also been starved. Cells lining the gut have died and not been replaced because of inadequate nutrient supply. The villi will have atrophied and the epithelial layers are thin and fragile, while digestive and absorptive capacities are severely limited.

When dogs and cats are fasting (either voluntarily or of necessity), they use body stores of fat and protein for energy. Whenever weight loss occurs, not only is adipose tissue reduced but lean body mass is also lost. This lean body mass loss is easily seen in reduction of skeletal muscle. The loss of protein from the internal tissues, e.g. heart and intestines, which accompanies it, is not immediately evident but is potentially more serious. Any animal showing signs of atrophy of the skeletal muscles is in urgent need of nutritional support.

This support must, however, be provided slowly; very small meals of highly digestible food should be given at regular intervals, the amount given being only slowly increased.

Although we encounter true starvation only rarely, most of us will be familiar with the undernourished stray dog which is presented at the surgery and put in a kennel until 'something is sorted out'. It is pathetically grateful for attention, and food is usually greeted with a feeble wag of the tail. Food is almost continually placed in front of it by a procession of staff who feel sorry for it, including those of us who should know better. The resultant diarrhoea does not find as many enthusiasts waiting to clean the kennel.

In a more severe case, overfeeding places a huge stress on the debilitated animal and may push one that is close to death over the edge, so resist the temptation to overfeed.

> Resist the temptation to overfeed.

The first step is to restore fluid levels, as many of these animals will show some degree of dehydration. A drip line may be necessary, otherwise very small amounts of fluid should be provided at frequent intervals. Electrolyte replacers can be used if tolerated.

At times of stress, animals revert to their nutritional heritage and as dogs and cats will use fats and protein for energy, carbohydrate should be used sparingly. A liquid or semi-liquid diet may be most appropriate. The food should be easily digested, although the limiting factor in utilization by the body is often not the digestibility of the food but rather the absorption of it. Small molecules can diffuse through the walls of the intestines but larger ones require active transport involving carrier proteins, which will have been reduced in numbers, so only small amounts of these larger molecules can be dealt with at any one time.

It is often recommended that feeding levels be built up over 3 days, feeding one-third of the daily requirement on day 1, two-thirds on day 2 and the full amount on day 3. This is only appropriate when food deprivation has been short term; long-standing deprivation will require more gradual increments. Each animal should be treated as an individual and its progression carefully monitored.

As it begins to recover it is appropriate to include pre- and probiotics to re-establish gut flora and encourage rebuilding of the gut walls. A change to a more 'normal' diet can also be instigated, but any dietary change must be made very gradually, bearing in mind the fragility of the system.

CRITICAL CARE NUTRITION

The above scenario is what perhaps most of us think of as 'starvation', but any illness or injury (including routine operations) carries with it the potential for protein energy malnutrition (PEM), an accelerated form of starvation which occurs when increased demands for protein and energy are aggravated by anorexia or inappetance, resulting in depletion of the body's protein and fat stores.

The body's initial response to illness or injury is to shut down systems to conserve limited resources: blood pressure drops, cardiac output is reduced and less oxygen is consumed. This is clinical shock, which is normally treated, and is known as the Ebb Phase. It is followed by the Flow or Hypermetabolic Phase, during which the body's defence and repair mechanisms are brought into play. This results in an increased demand for protein and energy and is less often treated, despite the likelihood of the animal being anorexic, perhaps because it is easy to imagine that, as the animal is apparently resting, it has less need for food.

In a normal healthy animal undergoing routine surgery, there is usually no need for any additional nutritional provision. Where illness is prolonged, injury is severe or either occur in an already debilitated animal, nutritional support will be required to prevent PEM developing.

Without nutritional support, the reduction in body stores of protein and energy can result in several adverse effects including:

- reduced immune responses leading to increased likelihood of sepsis
- delayed fracture and wound healing
- muscle weakness – skeletal muscle and also myocardium and muscles of the gastrointestinal tract, etc.
- anaemia.

If this catabolic state is allowed to continue, organ failure or even death may result.

Inappetant cats with chronic renal failure and a dog with a fractured jaw are obvious examples of animals needing nutritional support. Less obvious examples are the thin bitch spay normally fed on a cereal-based diet and the young cat spay who has been carrying a heavy flea burden. Both of these will benefit from an improved diet for 1–2 weeks after the operation, even more so if they can also receive the improved diet for a short while before undergoing surgery. (The normal proviso of dietary change taking place over 3–5 days still applies.)

Despite these examples, not all cases will need nutritional support, but any animal which has suffered rapid weight loss (10% or more within the previous 1–2 weeks) or has not eaten for 3 or more days, is likely to benefit from some degree of support. Debilitated animals and those with low body stores of fat or protein should also be carefully assessed for nutritional support.

Nutritional support should be introduced as soon as possible. Remember that once signs of skeletal muscle atrophy are apparent, nutrient deprivation changes will probably have also occurred in other tissues. Unless precluded by the illness or injury, support should be provided via the gut. Parenteral nutrition is expensive, time consuming, difficult to administer and allows the gut to atrophy which, in turn, presents problems when returning to enteral feeding.

The problem in these cases is often not providing food but ensuring that it is eaten.

Dehydration, if present, should be corrected and underlying problems addressed. Medical problems may indicate dietary change and physical problems will require adjustments in the way the animal is fed – a wired jaw may preclude solid food.

The increase in nutritional requirements comes at a time when the animal can often only be persuaded to eat small amounts, so the use of an energy-dense food is appropriate. Fat and protein will be more easily digested than carbohydrate and have the advantage of improving palatability, while fat increases the energy density. High biological value and ease of digestibility will ensure that as much of the food as possible is utilized by the body.

As with starvation, when the animal has not eaten for several days, feeding levels should be built up gradually and progress carefully monitored. If the animal is to receive medication in tablet form, it is better to administer these separately rather than crush them in food as this can increase the animal's suspicions and reduce the likelihood of the food being eaten.

Nutritional support will need to be provided for varying lengths of time depending on the severity of the illness or injury. Trauma cases will require support for between 2 and 12 weeks, but in the case of uncomplicated surgery, nutritional support for 10–14 days will probably be sufficient. Animals that have suffered from starvation may require support for up to 6 weeks and cancer patients may require long-term support, in many cases for the rest of their lives.

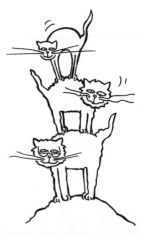

Fact

Fat and protein are more easily digested than carbohydrates.

Nutritional support

Trauma: 2–12 weeks
Surgery: 10–14 days
Starvation: up to 6 weeks
Cancer: long term

Nutrition and the immune system

The first line of defence in the body's attempt to ward off infection includes protective barriers such as the skin and intestinal mucosa. When these structures are weakened or damaged, the risk of infection is increased. The integrity of these barriers can be related to the level of nutrition, e.g. protein deficiency will weaken tissues. Other aspects of the immune system are also affected by the absence or insufficiency of nutrients, particularly certain vitamins and minerals.

Malnourished animals are therefore likely to have a compromised immune system and extra care should be taken with regard to hygiene, etc.

CANCER CACHEXIA

Cancer cachexia is a particular form of accelerated starvation, and protein energy malnutrition can be very severe in these cases, especially in those patients with aggressive, rapidly growing tumours. These animals have a greatly increased need for protein and energy to supply the tumour which has a continuous requirement for amino acids and energy. Unfortunately, at the same time the animal is often unable to take in extra nutrients, either because of the physical presence of the tumour or because the treatment the animal is receiving suppresses its appetite. In addition to this, products released by the body in the presence of tumours affect metabolic processes in the host animal, leading to either inefficient conversion of nutrients to energy or to excessive energy use.

The severity of cancer cachexia depends on the site of the neoplasm and on the individual, but in all cases, nutritional support will be required. In humans at least, maintaining bodyweight is known to improve the prognosis and it makes sense that an animal which avoids severe weight loss and all its implications for the body, is in better shape to fight the primary disease, particularly so when the immune responses are not suppressed by lack of protein.

Tumour tissue is an obligate glycolytic tissue relying on glucose as its energy source, unlike much of the body, which is able to use fat and protein for energy. A diet that is high in fat and protein but low in simple carbohydrates will provide energy to the body and meet increased protein demands while reducing the amount of energy available to the tumour cells. It will also, of course, have the added advantages of increased palatability and energy density. The amount fed will need to be carefully monitored and adjustments made as are appropriate for the animal's condition and progression of the disease. Small meals fed often will usually be more beneficial than larger, less frequent meals.

SKELETAL DISEASE

Although the nutritional requirements for correct bone growth and maintenance are well known, nutritionally-related skeletal disorders are still seen relatively often. It is usually young, growing animals that are affected, but adults are not exempt from these disorders.

Formation and maintenance of healthy bone requires a regular balanced supply of calcium and phosphorus, together with several vitamins and other minerals, energy and protein.

Calcium is essential in the body for many functions in addition to bone deposition, and the plasma concentrations are maintained within narrow margins by the hormones parathyroid (PTH) and calcitonin (CT) and by a derivative of vitamin D (DHC). Calcium inputs to the plasma are from the diet via the gut or from bones via resorption. Outputs are via bone deposition, losses through urine and faeces, and in pregnant or lactating animals, through fetal growth and milk production (see Figure 5.2). Any disruption in the mechanisms controlling the calcium plasma concentration, or excesses or deficiencies in the diet related to the calcium plasma levels, can lead to skeletal disease.

As calcium and phosphorus interrelate, the proportions of one to the other are important and the body will attempt to maintain the correct ratio between them. When dietary phosphorus is increased, more is absorbed from the gut and the concentration of phosphorus in plasma rises. Without a corresponding increase in calcium from the diet, this has the effect of decreasing calcium levels relative to phosphorus and calcium is drawn from the bones to balance the ratio. This is termed demineralization.

Dietary deficiencies

When a diet disproportionately high in muscle meat and organ tissue is fed, a relative calcium deficiency will occur because these foods contain sufficient phosphorus but inadequate amounts of calcium. The plasma concentration of phosphorus is raised relative to the calcium levels, leading to hypocalcaemia as outlined above. This leads to a reduction in bone mineralization and, at the same time, triggers a hormone response which attempts to restore the correct ratio between the two minerals. This stimulates increased absorption of calcium from the gut and resorption from the bones. As a result the organic matrix of the bone is still formed but is not adequately mineralized. In growing animals rickets develops (bowing of the long bones and enlarged epiphyses), while adults develop osteomalacia (bone softening). When the bones are sufficiently weakened, pathological fractures will occur. This is **nutritional secondary hyperparathyroidism**. This can occur in all breeds of dogs, in cats and also in cage birds and reptiles.

Calcium deficiency may also occur when absorption is inadequate, as in the presence of oxalate or phytate (phytic acid) which act as binding agents. Both of these are found in plants so the calcium in a vegetarian diet may not be readily available.

Phosphorus deficiency is rare in dogs and cats because manufactured foods normally contain sufficient amounts, but the addition of calcium supplements that do not contain phosphorus may lead to an imbalance in the diet, creating a relative phosphorus deficiency. Cereal diets contain phosphorus in the form of phytic acid, which is not readily available to carnivores, and which binds with calcium and magnesium to form phytin. This means that although levels of phosphorus and calcium in cereal diets may, on paper, be adequately high, in practice they are often insufficient. This is particularly so when vegetarian diets are fed to growing pups, those recovering from bone trauma or pregnant or lactating bitches.

Vitamin D deficiency is also rare in dogs and cats but may occasionally arise when home-made, or poor quality, cereal diets are fed. Vitamin D is required for both absorption of calcium from the gut and for resorption from bone, so a deficiency results in low plasma levels of calcium.

Dietary modification aims to:

- prevent further damage occurring
- repair damage already present whenever possible.

This is achieved by:

- restoring the correct ratio of calcium to phosphorus
- ensuring adequate levels of vitamin D.

A nutritionally balanced commercial food designed for growth should be fed. Supplementation should be avoided to prevent further upset in the mineral ratios.

Vitamins A and C and copper are also essential for skeletal growth and maintenance, but deficiencies are unlikely to occur when the animal is fed a balanced diet.

Only vegetables?!

Dietary excesses

Deficiencies are relatively easy to treat and correct but excesses cause more severe damage and are less easy to treat.

An excess of phosphorus will, as we have seen, lead to demineralization, but an excess of calcium absorbed from the gut causes hypercalcaemia which, in turn, leads to decreased resorption of calcium from the bones. The result is excess bone deposition which interferes with normal bone development and produces skeletal abnormalities. (It is thought that this may be a factor in the development of both hip dysplasia and wobbler syndrome.) Cartilage is affected as well as bone tissue. Disruption in the normal ossification process gives rise to thickened cartilage which is easily damaged; there is then the possibility of pieces breaking off and falling into the joint space, osteochondritis dissecans (OCD) which occurs most commonly in the distal condyles of the humerus and femur.

Excess calcium levels linked to excess energy is particularly a problem in puppies of large or giant breeds. The changes which occur are not readily reversible, so prevention is very important.

Dietary modification aims to:

- restore the correct ratio of calcium to phosphorus
- reduce energy levels.

Young animals should be fed a growth diet appropriate to the species, breed and age and a careful check kept on weight and condition. If signs of skeletal damage occur on this growth diet, the amount fed should be reduced to slow growth. This will not prevent the animal reaching its full adult size, but it will take longer to do so.

Excesses of vitamins A and D are particularly worrying as these vitamins are stored in the liver and the effects are cumulative, so that even small excesses can, over time, produce serious results. Excesses of both these vitamins will cause skeletal problems, the most well known being vitamin A excess in cats which causes postural changes in these animals. Owners who feed their cats large amounts of liver should be alerted to the potential danger of doing so.

Dietary modification aims to:

- remove the source of excess vitamins from the diet
- supply an appropriate balanced diet.

Prevention is more important than treatment, as the prognosis in many cases involving dietary excesses is guarded.

Most skeletal problems will occur in growing animals, so good dietary advice should be given to owners of puppies (particularly those of the most susceptible breeds) and kittens as early as possible.

Arthritis

Arthritis (inflammation of a joint) is a condition which is commonly seen in older dogs. Dietary supplements are now available, e.g. chondroitin and glucosamine, for use in animals suffering from this and other degenerative joint diseases. These supplements aim to slow progression of the disease and promote repair of damaged tissue where possible. In most cases they do appear to reduce pain and improve mobility, thus improving the animal's quality of life.

Many of these animals are overweight to a greater or lesser extent and, in these cases, one dietary modification which will help is adjustment of calorie intake to restore the animal to its ideal bodyweight. This will reduce strain on joints and encourage greater mobility.

NEUROMUSCULAR DISEASE

Neuromuscular disorders of dietary origin are linked with deficiencies of nutrients. Most are rare in dogs and cats but are potentially a problem when inadequately balanced home-made diets are fed. The commonest example is probably inadequate levels of protein in the diet, causing the animal to use its body stores with marked reduction in muscle mass and consequent muscle weakness. Other deficiencies involve the lack of certain vitamins and minerals.

Magnesium deficiency causes muscle weakness and a lack of thiamin (vitamin B_1) gives rise to central nervous system (CNS) signs. In the latter case the problem may not be inadequate amounts of thiamin in the diet, but the presence of the antivitamin thiaminase.

Niacin and riboflavin usually occur together, so a deficiency in one will indicate a deficiency in the other. They are both involved in energy metabolism, so a deficiency in either can result in a variety of abnormalities including muscle weakness and CNS symptoms. The cat, unlike most mammals, is unable to synthesize niacin from the amino acid trytophan, so requires a dietary source. However as this vitamin is found in large quantities in meat, problems are rare.

A deficiency in selenium and/or vitamin E can give rise to steatitis or yellow fat disease in cats. This causes necrosis of fat cells and the cat suffers pain and discomfort when moving, thus giving the incorrect impression that muscle or nerves are involved.

Dietary modification aims to:

- correct deficiencies
- restore correct function of muscle and nerves.

This is achieved by provision of a good-quality, balanced diet.

Neurological disorders may appear secondary to pathological fractures, and other skeletal abnormalities may cause pinching of nerves as they emerge from the spinal cord. In these cases the prognosis for the original skeletal disorder is more guarded.

DISORDERS OF THE INTEGUMENT

The integument is the tissue covering the body, the skin plus hair (or feathers) and nails or claws. The skin and hair condition is often a reflection of the general health of the animal for two reasons:

- underlying problems may disrupt vascular circulation or nutrient supply
- a sick animal is often disinclined to groom itself or may be physically unable to.

Healthy skin should be supple, appear clean and be without patches of reddened or moist tissue. It should be neither dry and scaly nor excessively greasy. The hair coat should be glossy and even, with no broken ends or thin or bald patches. It should have a texture and density appropriate to the breed.

As animals age the skin tends to become drier and lose its elasticity and the hair becomes less glossy, often loses pigment and the coat may be less thick than previously.

These changes are normal but other deviations from the normal condition may indicate underlying disorders.

There are only a limited number of ways in which the skin can react to deficiency, disease or irritant, so similar symptoms can appear for a variety of reasons – especially designed to challenge the dermatologists. As an example, miliary dermatitis commonly seen in the cat, is the skin's response to excessive licking by the cat's abrasive tongue, due to irritation of some kind. This irritation is often due to flea bites but is not confined to this cause.

Some skin conditions can be related to the animal's diet, namely dietary deficiencies or reactions due to food intolerance or hypersensitivity.

Dietary deficiencies

Although most nutrients have a role to play in the maintenance of healthy skin and hair, the main problems are associated with inadequate protein or deficiencies of vitamin A, zinc or fatty acids.

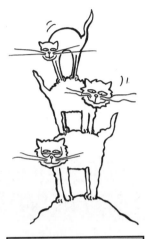

- Protein – up to 30% of the daily protein requirement is utilized by the body in the maintenance of normal skin and hair growth. Protein deficiency will therefore affect the integument producing abnormal keratinization of the skin and a poor, thin coat which lacks lustre and, in severe cases, will produce patchy alopecia. A relative shortage of protein may occur in bitches at the end of pregnancy or during lactation, when their diet fails to take into account their increased need for protein at these times. Puppies and kittens raised on an inadequate diet may also have a poor coat for the same reason.

  Long-term protein deficiency is rarely seen except in animals that are maintained on a very low protein diet because of some other unrelated problem, e.g. chronic renal failure.

- Vitamin A and zinc – most pet animals are now fed proprietary diets at least part of the time, and so absolute deficiencies are unlikely to occur. Relative deficiencies may arise because of the relationships between nutrients. A relative vitamin A deficiency may occur in animals on a fat-restricted diet or in those who have fat absorption problems. Young, growing animals or pregnant or lactating females are most at risk under these circumstances. Absorption of zinc is affected by other nutrients in the diet. Calcium, iron and copper all compete with zinc for the same absorption sites, so that an excess of any one of these can upset the absorption of the others. Phytates in the diet will bind with zinc, reducing or preventing absorption. This can be a problem when dogs are fed a poor-quality, cereal-based food.

- Essential fatty acids (EFAs) have both structural and biochemical roles in the skin and several skin conditions will respond to supplementation with EFAs. Animals who suffer from fat malabsorption and those with liver problems are obvious candidates for supplementation, but others without apparent internal disorders may also respond to EFA supplements. The response may take several weeks to become apparent and owners should be encouraged to continue with the supplement, when it has been recommended, for at least 6 weeks.

Fact

Most dietary problems are due to deficiencies of protein, vitamin A, zinc or fatty acids.

Proprietary foods normally contain adequate amounts of EFAs, but linoleic acid levels in dry foods may fall when the food is stored incorrectly.

Dietary modification aims to:

- reduce the symptoms
- repair the damage.

This is achieved by:

- restoring a correctly balanced diet
- supplementation when necessary.

Over-supplementation should be avoided, particularly in the case of vitamins and minerals, to prevent further upsets in the nutrient balance of the diet and to avoid excesses, which can be as damaging as deficiencies.

FOOD INTOLERANCE AND SENSITIVITY

These are often referred to as allergies and it may be useful here to remind ourselves of the difference between allergy, intolerance and sensitivity.

- Allergy – an allergy is a reaction which occurs when the body produces the allergy antibody, immunoglobulin E (IgE), in response to contact with a substance that is normally harmless. Once an allergy has developed, only a very small amount of allergen will produce a reaction. True allergies are rare.
- Intolerance – an intolerance occurs when the body cannot digest a particular substance. This is often due to a shortage of, or lack of, an enzyme that acts on that particular nutrient. Intolerances usually only cause problems when large amounts of the food are eaten.
- Sensitivity – this occurs when an existing medical problem is triggered or made worse by the ingestion of certain foods. The food is not the cause of the problem and the symptoms are not due to an allergic response. Skin problems are often multifactorial in cause and may remain in check while the combined effects remain below the pruritic threshold, i.e. the level at which irritation causes scratching. Sensitivity, which produces an exaggerated response to a particular food, may push the combined effects of several causes over this threshold and lead to the appearance of symptoms. Reduction of the effect of any one factor should reduce the total effect back below the threshold and thus resolve the symptoms.

EXCLUSION DIETS

When dietary intolerance or hypersensitivity is suspected in either skin or intestinal conditions, an exclusion diet may be recommended. The aim is to identify the particular product to which the body is reacting so that it can be avoided in future. There may, of course, be more than one product which triggers a reaction.

Proprietary exclusion diets are available and should be used if such a diet is required long term or for more than 3 weeks in immature animals, as they provide a fully balanced diet. Initially, however, home-made diets are often best.

The first step is to find foods which do not produce a reaction, after which other products can be introduced one by one, to study their effect on the body. The dietary trial should proceed in an ordered way if it is to be of value.

- The home-made diet should consist of those ingredients that are either totally new to the animal or have not been eaten by the animal in the past month.
- The diet should contain as few ingredients as possible to ensure a true trial. It should consist of one animal protein, e.g. chicken, lamb or fish, one carbohydrate, e.g. boiled rice or potato, and water. No other food should be fed during the trial and no treats given.
- The diet should be fed for a minimum of 3 weeks. Occasionally a response will show before this time. If no response occurs in 3 weeks, it should be continued for up to 10 weeks before a dietary intolerance or sensitivity is ruled out.
- When the condition goes into remission, the original food may be reintroduced to help determine whether the response is coincidental or whether an intolerance or sensitivity exists.
- If a relapse does occur when the original food is fed, intolerance or sensitivity is a high probability and the animal should be returned to the home-made diet.
- If remission occurs again, intolerance or sensitivity is confirmed.
- Challenge studies can now take place to try to identify the particular product causing the problem. Individual products are added to the home-made diet and the response is monitored. It should then be possible to construct a balanced diet for long-term use, avoiding those products which produce a response in the body.

An alternative at this point is to introduce a commercially-prepared diet containing protein from only one or two sources (most intolerances and sensitivities are reactions to proteins). If this is accepted and no relapse occurs, the diet can be fed for life. Most home-made elimination diets are nutritionally inadequate to a greater or lesser degree and are not therefore recommended for long-term use.

Some owners may prefer to go directly to the commercial exclusion diet and maintain their pet on that, provided the symptoms are resolved.

CARDIOVASCULAR DISEASE

Cardiovascular disease occurs in both dogs and cats but is seen most often in dogs.

A small percentage of animals have congenital heart disease but most cases will develop as the animal ages. Of those animals that develop heart disease, a high percentage of cases will progress to heart failure, i.e. the inability of the heart to pump enough blood to supply the body tissues with sufficient oxygen and nutrients. Heart failure may be of acute onset with sudden cardiac arrest, but more often develops slowly when impaired pumping ability is associated with abnormal fluid retention; this is congestive heart failure (CHF). Although there are many causes of heart failure in the dog, the two commonest are chronic valvular disease and dilated cardiomyopathy.

- Chronic valvular disease occurs when a valve in the heart (usually the mitral valve but sometimes the tricuspid valve) degenerates, and no longer forms an effective seal. When the mitral valve is affected, blood will leak back through to the atrium as the left ventricle contracts, reducing the output to the aorta.
- Dilated cardiomyopathy occurs when contraction of the heart muscle (myocardium) is reduced. The muscle becomes slack and the atria and ventricles enlarge. Weaker contractions mean less blood is pumped and the output to the body is again reduced.

The frequency with which both these conditions appear increases with age. Chronic valvular disease is most common in small breeds, whereas dilated cardiomyopathy is largely restricted to large and giant breeds.

A reduction in output from the heart triggers compensatory responses from the body which result

> ### Fact
> The two most common causes of heart failure in the dog are chronic valvular disease and dilated cardiomyopathy.

in an increase in heart rate and strength of contractions, an increase in the volume of circulating blood and a constriction of peripheral vessels, not only in the skin but also in gut, spleen and kidney. These compensatory mechanisms unfortunately can have an adverse effect on the body.

The increased rate and strength of contraction can further damage the heart and excess water retention leads to congestion in the lungs and other organs. Oedema develops and is increased by the inability of fluid to return to the circulation from the tissues because of the constriction of peripheral vessels.

This constriction also has adverse effects on the efficiency of other organs, interfering with the uptake of nutrients from the gut and affecting the liver and kidneys. When heart failure occurs in elderly animals, the function of these organs may already be impaired and will be worsened by the compensatory mechanisms. It is likely that animals with heart disease will have other concurrent problems, which must be considered when dietary advice is given.

Dilated cardiomyopathy can occur in cats but has been linked in this instance to a long term deficiency of taurine in the diet. Since the addition of this amino acid to commercial cat foods, the incidence of the condition in cats has fallen.

In those animals predisposed to heart disease, being overweight increases the chances of it developing, so some CHF patients will be obese. Other animals will be underweight, partly because these cases are often anorexic, but also because of malabsorption and altered metabolism of protein and fat leading to noticeable muscle wastage.

Dietary modification aims to:

- reduce pulmonary oedema and ascites
- restore the animal to normal body weight
- maintain lean body mass
- provide support for other organs which may be compromised.

To achieve this the diet should:

- have reduced sodium and chloride levels, although the degree of restriction will depend on the drug therapy being used
- have potassium levels appropriate to the drug therapy used
- have increased levels of the B complex vitamins
- have increased levels of taurine, helpful to dogs as well as essential for cats
- have moderate levels of high biological value protein

- have a calorie density appropriate to the condition of the animal.

It is necessary to consider the drugs used to treat cardiovascular disease because of the effects they have on the body; for example:

- ACE inhibitors are vasodilators and also reduce aldosterone levels. This reduces the retention of sodium and the excretion of potassium.
- Digoxin improves heart muscle contraction and has no direct effect on dietary requirements.
- Diuretics – frusemide increases the excretion of sodium, potassium and magnesium.

The benefits of restricting salt levels early in the course of heart disease are subject to much debate. The main benefit would seem to be accustoming the animal to a less appetizing diet. Salt is usually added to foods to improve palatability and the reduction of salt levels is therefore believed to reduce comparable palatability. Many animals, as cardiovascular disease progresses, become anorexic and palatability then becomes a matter of concern. If these animals have previously become accustomed to lower palatability levels, low sodium diets will be more readily accepted. Some proprietary diets have non-salt products added to improve palatability while allowing sodium and chlorine levels to be reduced.

In the later stages, home-made diets are often more acceptable to the animal than commercially prepared ones, but care must be taken to avoid foods which have naturally high salt levels (Table 7.1). Adding

Table 7.1 Foods containing high levels of salt

bacon	offal
bread	processed meats
breakfast cereals	smoked meat and fish
cheese	tinned fish in brine
egg	

These are mainly 'human' foods. Owners should preferably use unprocessed meats, e.g. chicken, turkey and rabbit, and basic carbohydrate foods, e.g. rice, pasta and potatoes.

gravy or stock cubes should be avoided as these usually contain high salt levels. It is sometimes recommended that distilled water is offered to avoid the possibility of high sodium levels in the local water supply but this may not be acceptable to the animal and is probably unnecessary in most places.

Hypertension

In the past, blood pressure has not been routinely measured in dogs and cats but with the increasing availability of reliable equipment, these measurements will become more common. At present there is little information on this problem in the pet population but this could change in the near future as the level of incidence is discovered.

Currently hypertension is thought to occur chiefly as a secondary condition, arising when another disease process affects the body's ability to maintain blood pressure, e.g. primary cardiac disease causing sodium retention, renal disease or Cushing's disease.

Current dietary recommendations involve addressing the underlying causes but new recommendations are likely to be made as knowledge and understanding of the problem increases.

THE DIGESTIVE SYSTEM

Other parts of the body are affected by the chemical effects of food, but the gastrointestinal tract is affected by both the chemical and mechanical aspects of the food eaten. It is necessary, therefore, to consider both the composition of food and its physical characteristics when choosing what to feed, particularly in relation to the upper regions of the digestive system.

Teeth

The correct calcium to phosphorus ratio is important in the young animal to ensure correct development of the teeth but, thereafter, the effects of food on the teeth is largely mechanical. Soft foods tend to cling to the teeth, encouraging the build up of plaque which, if not removed, becomes mineralized to form calculus (tartar) with consequent inflammation of the gums and eventually peridontitis. Dry foods are more abrasive and help remove plaque from the teeth. For those animals that seem to have a preference for moist foods, replacing one-third of the daily ration with dry food is a helpful compromise.

In the wild, tearing and chewing fresh prey cleans the teeth in a way that commercial foods cannot replicate, but providing treats which need to be chewed will help with plaque removal. When such chews are given, an appropriate reduction should be made in the main diet to allow for the extra calories contained in the treat. Proprietary dry foods are also available with a texture designed to scrape plaque from the teeth. These are complete foods and can be fed either on their own (when their effect is greatest) or in conjunction with another food.

Oesophagus

Regurgitation, the passive reflux of undigested food, usually occurs immediately after swallowing, but can be delayed for quite long periods and may be mistakenly reported by the owner as vomiting. It is important to differentiate between the two, as regurgitation indicates a problem within the posterior pharynx or oesophagus, whereas vomiting occurs when the problem is located in the stomach or small intestines.

Regurgitation may indicate the presence of a foreign body, but may also occur for a variety of reasons, including pharyngitis/oesophagitis and megaoesophagus.

- Pharyngitis/oesophagitis can be caused by trauma or infection, but in either case is likely to cause pain on swallowing and the animal is often reluctant to eat for this reason. In severe cases it may be necessary to withhold food for 2–3 days or to instigate tube feeding. In most cases, very soft food should be fed in several small meals. Canned food can be mashed or liquidized with additional water, or semi-liquid or liquid convalescent diets can be offered. A gradual return to the animal's normal food can be made as soon as the problem is resolved.
- Megaoesophagus occurs when the oesophagus fails to contract and food is no longer propelled backwards to the stomach. It will either be returned immediately or may pool in the oesophagus for some time before being regurgitated. In these cases the oesophagus becomes dilated and is able to hold quite large amounts of food. It may occur secondary to myasthenia gravis.

Dietary modification (and method of feeding) aims to:

- minimize regurgitation and reduce risk of secondary aspiration
- provide adequate nutrition.

> **Definition**
>
> Regurgitation is the passive reflux of undigested food.

Dry foods are often best for animals with mega-oesophagus as these seem to stimulate the oesophagus better than softer foods and may reduce the risk of aspiration pneumonia. All animals are, however, individuals and some will do better on soft foods. Trial and error will indicate which is best for each case. Whichever type of food is chosen, it should be nutrient-dense, to reduce the amount which needs to be fed, appropriate to the age of the animal and be easily digestible. The daily ration should be split into a minimum of three equal portions and fed at regular intervals.

The animal should not have to bend its head to eat and should be trained to eat from a position that raises the head and neck, thus enabling gravity to assist in moving food down to the stomach. Bowls can be placed on worktops, stairs, stools or specially made stands. Water also needs to be available in the elevated position.

Gastric dilation-volvulus

This is another disorder in which the method and timing of feeding is of equal or more importance, than the type of diet fed.

Gastric dilation-volvulus (GD-V) is a serious and potentially fatal condition which frequently requires surgery. The stomach dilates rapidly with food, fluid or gas from swallowed air or fermentation of the food and the swollen stomach may then rotate trapping the stomach contents. Gastric ulceration and haemorrhage, together with hypovolaemic shock, severe electrolyte disturbances and the development of cardiac arrhythmias, are all complications of this syndrome which add to its severity.

It is important to relieve the tension on the stomach as quickly as possible. Where twisting (volvulus) has not occurred, passing a stomach tube will release the gases, but when volvulus has taken place, immediate surgery is necessary.

The cause is unknown but there seem to be several risk factors involved:

- breed – large, deep-chested breeds (e.g. German Shepherd Dogs, Great Danes, St Bernards, Dobermanns, Irish Setters and Bassets) seem to be predisposed to GD-V
- age – older dogs are more susceptible
- over-eating and over-drinking followed by exercise
- aerophagia

- gastric fermentation
- previous gastric trauma.

It was thought that cereal-based foods fed dry were a predisposing factor but this is not necessarily the case. Many large breed dogs are fed this type of diet for ease and cost reasons without developing GD-V. One method of feeding this type of diet may, however, be a risk factor. Cereal-based diets are often of low digestibility and are low in calories, so correspondingly large amounts have to be eaten to satisfy the dog's nutritional requirements. When this amount is fed in one meal per day, the stomach enlarges over time and becomes more muscular. This leads to delayed gastric emptying and stretching of the gastrohepatic ligament, weakening it and making it easier for the stomach to twist.

Although the causes of GD-V are not fully understood, the following dietary advice is usually given in the hope of preventing recurrence of the problem:

- feed a highly digestible, low-fat, low-residue diet to encourage rapid gastric emptying
- calorie density should be as high is as compatible with the above recommendations to reduce the volume which needs to be fed
- divide the daily ration into a minimum of three equal portions
- avoid exercise or excitement before and after feeding
- feed away from other animals to remove the risk of competitive eating – gulping food increases the amount of air swallowed
- water should be provided on a 'little and often' basis.

The gastrointestinal tract has three functions directly related to the food ingested:

- motility – the grinding of food to smaller particles, mixing and transport of ingesta
- secretion – hormones and enzymes to stimulate and assist digestion plus fluids and electrolytes secreted into the lumen of the gut
- digestion – the absorption of ingested materials, together with resorption of fluids and electrolytes.

The complexities and interactions of these functions, together with the ingestion of substances of questionable origin, lend themselves to the possibility of many dysfunctional and disease states developing. Many of these problems will give rise to one or both of the two main clinical signs associated with the gastrointestinal tract – vomiting and diarrhoea.

Vomiting

Vomiting, which should not be confused with regurgitation, is defined as the forcible ejection of the partially digested contents of the stomach and/or the proximal duodenum, through the mouth. Vomiting is usually accompanied by rhythmic contractions of the abdomen. It may be acute or chronic.

> **Definition**
>
> Vomiting is the forcible ejection of the partially digested contents of the stomach and/or the proximal duodenum through the mouth.

- In the dog, acute vomiting is usually associated with injudicious eating, either of contaminated material or ingestion of too large quantities resulting in gastric distension. These problems occur much less frequently in cats, as they are more particular in their choice of food and tend to be less greedy, although nibbling toxic household plants is one problem which does occur in cats, particularly kittens.
- Chronic vomiting is more often associated with underlying problems. Gastric stasis will, over time, lead to gastric distension even when normal amounts of food are eaten. Foreign bodies in the stomach or small intestines forming total or partial blockages, infections, tumours and parasites are a few examples of possible problems.

Vomiting may also be caused by factors outside the gastrointestinal tract, e.g. travel sickness caused by stimulation of the cerebellum or uraemia or ketosis arising as a result of disease elsewhere in the body.

The timing of vomiting, in relation to the time of feeding and the appearance of the vomit, will give clues as to the cause; however, nutritional management of the vomiting animal is broadly similar regardless of cause.

When a diagnosis has been made and treatment for the underlying cause initiated if necessary, **dietary modification aims to**:

- restore fluid and electrolyte balance
- enable the animal to return to its normal diet.

To achieve this it is necessary to:

- replace lost fluids, either orally or with intravenous fluids
  - orally: water or electrolyte solution given little and often (every 15–30 minutes if possible). Some animals dislike the taste of electrolyte solutions and will need active encouragement to take them
  - intravenous fluids: used when oral fluids are not tolerated or when total gastric rest is desired
- introduce a bland diet, feeding little and often (five to six times daily) and gradually build up the

quantities given over a period of 3 days. Suitable home-made diets use one part by weight protein with two parts by weight of carbohydrate for dogs and equal parts by weight of protein and carbohydrate for cats (weights are cooked weights). Scrambled egg, cottage cheese, boiled chicken, boiled rice (baby rice cereal for cats) are all suitable foods. When boiling chicken, the water used should be saved and the rice cooked in it to improve palatability. Proprietary bland diets are also available.

- reintroduce the normal diet gradually. Sudden changes in diet are themselves a cause of vomiting (and diarrhoea), so the changeover should take place over a minimum of 3 days.

If vomiting returns when the animal is back on its normal diet, dietary management of the case needs to be reviewed.

In cases of chronic gastritis, the animal may need to be maintained on a diet which is low in protein (protein stimulates the secretion of gastric acid) and fat (fat delays stomach emptying) and relatively high in carbohydrate.

Some otherwise healthy, small nervous dogs have a tendency to vomit in the morning (bilious vomiting syndrome). Bland diets are recommended for these dogs, with one-third of the daily ration fed in the morning and two-thirds in the evening.

Diarrhoea

Diarrhoea is defined as the rapid movement of faecal material through the intestines producing loose or liquid stools. The result is reduced absorption of water, electrolytes and nutrients. The loss of water and electrolytes leads to dehydration and acidosis. Diarrhoea can be either acute or chronic.

- Acute diarrhoea is most often due to irritation of the gut mucosa by infections, toxins or parasites and may, if not adequately treated, develop into chronic diarrhoea.
- Chronic diarrhoea has many other causes, including small intestine bacterial overgrowth (SIBO), inflammatory bowel disease and neoplasia. To some extent nutritional management of diarrhoea will depend on its origin, so it is helpful to be able to differentiate between diarrhoea arising in the small intestine and that arising in the large intestine (Table 7.2).

The aim with chronic diarrhoea should, whenever possible, be to determine the underlying cause. Care-

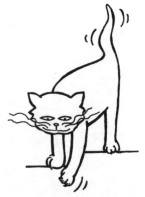

Definition

Diarrhoea is defined as the rapid movement of faecal material through the intestines producing loose or liquid stools.

Table 7.2 Differentiation of diarrhoeas

Clinical sign	Small intestine	Large intestine
Frequency and timing	Large volumes infrequently	Small volumes frequently
Tenesmus (ineffectual and painful straining)	Little or none	Often seen (sometimes mistaken by owner as constipation)
Discomfort	Little or none	Often present
Losing weight	Yes	No
Passing blood	Dark	Fresh
Mucoid	No	Yes
Fat or undigested food	May be present	Absent

ful questioning of the owner and examination of a faecal sample will give a broad indication as to possible causes. More specific tests may lead to a firm diagnosis but sadly many cases are classed as idiopathic – having no known cause.

Flotation tests and microscopic examination of faecal samples may indicate the presence of parasites but diarrhoea, like vomiting, may be the result of disease elsewhere in the body and the value of routine biochemistry and haematology results should not be overlooked.

Specific blood tests used in the diagnosis of gastrointestinal disorders include:

- trypsin-like immunoreactivity (TLI) test
- folate
- cobalamin.

TLI – trypsinogen, the precursor of trypsin, is secreted exclusively by the pancreas and the TLI test is used to monitor the level of pancreatic enzymes in the blood. Little or no trypsin-like activity is an indication that there is insufficient production of enzymes by the pancreas. On the other hand, high levels will indicate a diagnosis of pancreatitis if amylase and lipase are also high.

Serum folate and cobalamin – folate (or folic acid) and cobalamin are vitamins belonging to the B group and in proprietary foods are normally present in amounts sufficient to prevent a dietary deficiency. Low serum levels are therefore an indication of intestinal dysfunction.

Folate is absorbed in the proximal small intestine and cobalamin in the distal small intestine. Low serum levels of folate may indicate malabsorption in the proximal small intestine and low serum levels of cobalamin, malabsorption in the distal section. Low levels of both indicate malabsorption throughout the small intestine.

Bacteria present in the gut produce folic acid and use cobalamin for their own metabolism. When bacterial numbers increase, the amount of folic acid produced is increased and the amount of cobalamin available to the animal is decreased. These changes are reflected in the serum levels and a high folate reading linked with a low cobalamin reading is indicative of small intestine bacterial overgrowth.

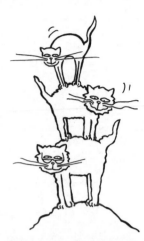

Radiographic or ultrasound scans may also be carried out. Biopsies can be taken and endoscopic examination is increasingly utilized in pursuit of a diagnosis.

> **Fact**
> High folate and low cobalamin = too many bacteria in the small intestine.

Acute diarrhoea

Acute diarrhoea will usually respond with 24–48 hours' starvation. Access to fluids should be allowed during this time to counteract dehydration and electrolyte imbalance. If the animal will accept electrolyte solutions these should be used, otherwise provide water (but not milk). After 24 or 48 hours a bland, easily digested food should be introduced and management continued as for vomiting cases. Very young animals should not be starved or at most for only a few hours. Medical intervention will probably be required much earlier than in adults and all such cases should be seen and assessed by a vet without undue delay.

Chronic diarrhoea

Two major causes of chronic diarrhoea are food and inflammation.

Food-related causes

As already stated, sudden changes in diet can lead to vomiting and diarrhoea. Sometimes the owner, seeing this as a side effect to the new food, will change the diet several times over a short period and very often this results in chronic diarrhoea. Different foods require the body to produce a different range of

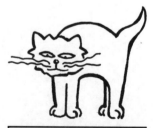

> **NB!**
> Too frequent changes of diet lead to chronic diarrhoea.

enzymes to digest them. This enzyme mix can normally only be changed slowly. When the mix of enzymes present is inadequate to digest the new food, digestion and absorption is reduced, leaving food particles within the intestines. These nutrients draw fluid into the gut through osmosis; the resultant diarrhoea is termed 'osmotic diarrhoea' and is commonly seen.

Management of osmotic diarrhoea is similar to the management of acute cases as diarrhoea ceases when the animal is starved. Once the animal is stable on an appropriate diet, the owner should be advised to stick with that diet and not make changes. When changes do become necessary, changeover should take place gradually over a period of 5–7 days.

Vomiting and diarrhoea can be caused by dietary hypersensitivity and intolerance. Sometimes the connection between a particular food and disorders of the gastrointestinal tract is very clear, other cases may involve the use of exclusion diets to determine the problem item. The protocol for this has already been outlined in the section dealing with skin conditions.

Gluten-sensitive enteropathy

A specific hypersensitivity which occurs chiefly, but not solely, in Irish Setters, is gluten-sensitive enteropathy. Affected animals are unable to digest gluten, resulting in diarrhoea, and either failure to gain weight or weight loss. Clinical signs often first become apparent around 6 months of age. Confirmation of gluten sensitivity means that the animal will need to be maintained on a gluten-free diet for life.

Inflammatory causes

Another common cause of chronic diarrhoea in both cats and dogs is inflammation, which interferes with normal digestion and absorption. This malabsorption and consequent lack of nutrients may produce clinical signs in other body systems, e.g. poor mineral and vitamin uptake may lead to poor skin and coat condition. Weight loss can be a problem in severe cases.

Inflammation may arise from infection, dietary intolerance, immune-mediated disorders, parasites or bacterial overgrowth and can occur throughout the small or large intestines. Inflammation of the small intestine has the greatest effect because it is here that absorption of nutrients takes place.

Regardless of cause, inflammatory disorders affecting the small intestine are often grouped together and termed inflammatory bowel disease (IBD).

Drug therapy will often be required but dietary management plays an important role in the treatment of all inflammatory bowel conditions.

Dietary modification for all cases of IBD aims to:

- reduce inflammation
- reverse intestinal change and restore normal function.

The underlying cause, if known, will suggest the most appropriate diet, but when cases of idiopathic origin are involved, the correct diet may only be achieved by trial and error. In the absence of a firm diagnosis, malabsorption as the most serious consequence should be addressed first.

A suitable diet is bland, non-irritant, highly digestible and avoids products known to cause diarrhoea such as gluten (rice is gluten free) and lactose. Low fibre content will ensure that residues are kept to the minimum. Levels of vitamins, particularly B complex vitamins, and some minerals (e.g. zinc), should be increased to compensate for deceased absorption. Common sense should suggest feeding little and often.

The above bland diet, if it consists of one protein and one carbohydrate, is also appropriate for suspected cases of dietary intolerance.

Animals with SIBO may have impaired fat digestion and absorption. Bacteria break down the bile salts, interfering with micelle formation and reducing fat digestibility. Excess fatty acids and bile salt residues in the bowel stimulate excess secretion of fluids into the gut and 'secretory diarrhoea' is produced.

Unfortunately, reducing the fat content reduces the calorie density of the diet and to compensate for this, medium-chain triglycerides (MCTs) may be added to diets for dogs. These are hydrolysed more efficiently and are absorbed into the portal circulation rather than the lymphatics. They must, however, be used with care in dogs, and not at all in cats. MCTs can be used to provide up to a fifth to one-quarter of the dog's daily calorie requirement; levels above this may cause anorexia and vomiting. Cats are in danger of developing hepatic lipidosis if fed MCTs. Cats do better on a diet containing reasonably high amounts of

To recap

Do not feed cats medium-chain triglycerides (MCTs) as they may develop hepatic lipidosis.

highly digestible fat. In this species low-fat diets may actually worsen the diarrhoea.

Medium-chain triglycerides are also of use when lymphatic drainage from the gut fails. As the lacteals form the main route of absorption for fatty acids, failure of the lymph drainage results in severely restricted fat absorption. A low-fat diet supplemented with MCTs will supply calories but, as stated before, must be used with care.

Lymphangiectasia

Lymphangiectasia is a condition in which lymphatic vessels become dilated and congested and lymph leaks out into the lumen of the gut. It can occur as a congenital condition but more often is present secondary to other diseases. As lymph contains both albumen and globulin, this condition results in loss of protein and is classed as a 'protein-losing enteropathy'.

Dietary modification aims to:

- provide moderate amounts of good-quality, highly digestible protein
- contain low fat levels but have added MCTs
- be high in fibre.

Protein-losing enteropathies may be the end result of many other chronic gastrointestinal problems, and symptoms include weight loss and poor condition as well as chronic diarrhoea. Treatment and dietary management of these enteropathies will depend on the underlying cause.

Colitis

Colitis (inflammation of the colon) is one of the commonest causes of diarrhoea in dogs. It also occurs in cats but less often. The condition has many causes, including stress, and careful questioning of the owner may point to this as the main cause. If stress can be modified or avoided, colitis may resolve without further intervention.

Colitis is characterized by the presence of mucus covering the faeces (owners often describe it as slime) and fresh blood, a fact that often prompts the owner to ring for advice earlier than in other cases of diarrhoea. The presence of mucus and fresh blood is not, however, restricted to colitis and when these symptoms occur, the animal should be fully checked by a vet.

Mild cases may be treated by diet alone, but more severe cases will require medical intervention.

As colitis has many causes, different cases will respond to different diets. When the cause is not easily determined the correct diet may, yet again, be a case of trial and error.

Dietary modification can take the form of:

- high-fibre diets – the presence of fibre will normalize the transit time and bind faecal water. Fermentable fibre will modify the strains and numbers of gut bacteria
- low-fibre, highly digestible diets (as for other forms of IBD) – low residues reduce the amount of unabsorbed food entering the colon. Highly digestible foods tend to reduce the number of bacteria in the colon
- hypoallergenic diets – to be used when dietary intolerance or hypersensitivity is suspected as the underlying cause.

In common with other causes of diarrhoea, it is usually recommended that the animal be starved for 24 hours before starting dietary treatment and that the daily ration of food is divided into two, three or four portions, at least in the initial stages of treatment.

If clinical signs are not controlled or there are frequent relapses, changing to another option should be tried. Resolution is complicated by the fact that colitis tends to appear spasmodically, with intervals of normality between bouts. The difficulty is knowing whether this normality is due to the pattern of the disease or to the treatment instigated.

When advising owners it is best to explain fully the various options of dietary management at the outset, as differing methods can appear contradictory and may lead to confusion.

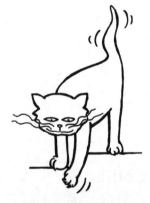

Constipation

Constipation occurs when the gut transit time is prolonged, resulting in hard, dry faeces which the animal is either unable to pass or has difficulty in doing so. The longer these hard, dry faeces remain in the rectum, the harder they become and then form an impacted mass. At times, very soft, watery faeces may be passed round this faecal impaction and this is termed 'obstipation'.

As with most gastrointestinal problems, there is no single cause. Factors involved range from ingestion of bones, hair or fur, through obstruction or constriction and neurological problems, to lack of exercise. Any condition which causes pain in the lower bowel or which interferes with the animal adopting its normal posture for defecation, can also lead to constipation.

Treatment involves:

- administering enemas to remove the build up of faeces
- determining and treating the underlying cause where possible
- instigating dietary management.

Dietary modification aims to:

- produce a soft but formed stool
- encourage regular defecation.

High-fibre diets increase faecal volume and increase the water content of faeces, softening the stool. Insoluble, poorly fermentable fibres are more effective in these respects than soluble, more highly ferment-able fibres. The increased bulk stimulates the large bowel to contract more efficiently, improving transit time and encouraging regular evacuation. The fibre may be incorporated as an integral part of the diet or may be added to the usual diet in the form of bran or other bulk-forming agents.

Dogs suffering from constipation should not be given bones, and cats which regularly catch and eat birds or small mammals should be encouraged to drink so that the contents of the large bowel do not become too dry. Both dogs and cats should be encouraged to exercise more.

Attention should also be paid to the animal's environment. Cats often prefer privacy and a clean litter tray; the absence of these may lead to retention of faeces. Some dogs will not pass faeces when on a lead or will only do so on certain surfaces (e.g. grass). This can cause problems when exercising hospitalized dogs; access to a safe run should be provided if possible.

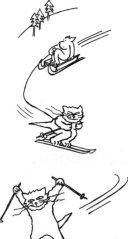

Exercise is good

Flatulence

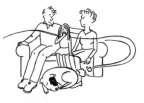

Flatulence is not noticeably a problem for pets but it is a problem for owners, their family and friends. Flatulence is chiefly a problem in dogs and is caused by excessive amounts of gas in the intestines. This excess may be due to swallowed air (aerophagia) or gas produced through bacterial fermentation of food.

Air is swallowed while eating or during panting and seems to be excessive in brachycephalic dogs. Animals that eat quickly, gulping their food, are also likely to swallow large amounts of air. Bacterial fermentation of poorly digestible carbohydrates or high-fibre diets is responsible for the production of large quantities of gas. Conditions which cause malabsorption allow excess amounts of undigested food to reach the colon where bacterial fermentation produces excess gas. The gases responsible for the unpleasant odours include ammonia and hydrogen sulphide. These normally form only a small proportion of the gas produced but certain foods will increase the levels of these gases with a subsequent rise in unpleasantness.

Dietary modification aims to:

- control aerophagia – feed little and often in a quiet area. Avoid competition from other animals
- use a high-quality, low-fat, low-residue diet
- avoid high-fibre diets, legumes, brassicas, potato, wheat and high-protein diets.

In the past, the addition of charcoal in the form of biscuits or as a powder has been recommended to absorb the gases, and in some cases this does appear to help. It is worth a try when other methods fail.

Borborygmus is a rumbling sound produced by the movement of gases through the gut, with the same causes and dietary management as flatulence.

Copraphagy

Another problem causing distress to dog owners is copraphagy, the ingestion of faeces. It is rarely a sign of dietary insufficiency and is more often a bad habit due to a depraved appetite (or pica). To some extent it is normal behaviour for bitches, which clean their pups and eat their faeces to keep the nest clean. If there is a clinical cause, exocrine pancreatic insufficiency is the most likely candidate. The main danger to the dog is the transmission of parasites.

Dietary modification should provide a highly digestible, energy-dense and low-residue diet, although in some cases higher fibre content has proved more effective.

When the animal concerned is eating its own faeces, the addition of pineapple juice to the diet is claimed to make the stools less palatable. Some proprietary foods are now available which contain additives that have the same effect.

Clearing away faeces promptly would seem to be a simpler and very effective way of preventing this problem.

> **Clinical tip**
>
> When an animal is eating its own faeces, the addition of pineapple juice to the diet is claimed to make the stools less palatable.

THE PANCREAS

The pancreas has both endocrine and exocrine functions (Figure 7.2). The endocrine secretions consist of hormones produced by the islets of Langerhans distributed throughout the pancreas. Disorders of the endocrine pancreas are covered in the section dealing with endocrine disorders.

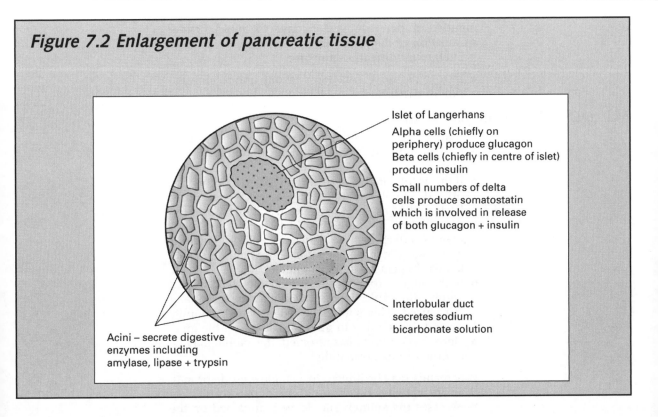

Figure 7.2 Enlargement of pancreatic tissue

Islet of Langerhans

Alpha cells (chiefly on periphery) produce glucagon
Beta cells (chiefly in centre of islet) produce insulin

Small numbers of delta cells produce somatostatin which is involved in release of both glucagon + insulin

Interlobular duct secretes sodium bicarbonate solution

Acini – secrete digestive enzymes including amylase, lipase + trypsin

Acute pancreatitis

The exocrine secretions, the pancreatic juice, include sodium bicarbonate to neutralize the acidity of the gastric contents, and digestive enzymes. These enzymes, amylase, lipase, trypsin and other proteolytic enzymes, are secreted in their inactive forms and empty into the duodenum where they are activated by a variety of mechanisms. There are several protective mechanisms which prevent the inactive enzymes becoming active while still in the pancreas, but occasionally these mechanisms fail and activated enzymes start to digest the pancreatic tissue. This causes severe damage and stimulates the production of further enzymes. Protease inhibitors in the pancreas are activated and bind with trypsin but this process can be overwhelmed and then the proteases can cause systemic damage. The stomach, small intestine and distal colon may all be affected, together with the liver and kidneys.

Drug therapy will be required, the amount depending on the extent of enzyme activation and tissue damage. Initially intravenous fluids will be required to restore fluid and electrolyte balance and it is essential that the animal has neither food nor fluid by

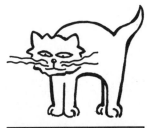

NB!

In cases of pancreatitis, nothing should be given by mouth for 3–5 days.

mouth (nil per os) for 3–5 days to avoid further stimulation of the pancreas.

Dietary modification aims to:

- restore digestive function without undue stimulation of the pancreas.

Management of acute pancreatitis

- If after 3 days vomiting has ceased, oral fluids may be reintroduced; small, frequent amounts for 2–3 days.
- If this is tolerated, a high-carbohydrate food may be offered, small amounts three to six times daily. Pasta, boiled rice or potato are all suitable. Carbohydrate supplies calories and has a minimal stimulatory effect on the pancreas. (Pasta contains gluten so should not be fed to those animals with a known hypersensitivity to gluten.)
- If the high-carbohydrate diet is tolerated, then a highly digestible, low-fat diet may be gradually introduced. This should be fed in small amounts several times a day to minimize stress on the gut.
- Once the condition has resolved, the animal may be returned to its normal diet.

Pancreatitis may be limited to a single episode or may recur repeatedly, becoming chronic pancreatitis. In these cases the animals should be maintained on the highly digestible, low-fat diet for life. Repeated bouts of pacreatitis can cause permanent damage within the pancreas and result in exocrine pancreatic insufficiency (EPI).

Exocrine pancreatic insufficiency

This is a condition which, as stated above, may occur as a result of chronic pancreatitis or as a congenital disorder, particularly in German Shepherd dogs. It is rare in cats.

Since atrophy of the acini (or in the case of pancreatitis, irreparable damage) is involved, treatment when required must be continued for life. The affected animal is unable to digest the food it eats and so is often very thin, in poor condition and has chronic diarrhoea.

Dietary modification aims to:

- replace the 'lost' enzymes
- restore bodyweight and condition
- maintain the animal on an appropriate diet.

Management of EPI

- Feed a highly digestible, low-fat diet twice daily. The calorie requirement should be based on the animal's current weight. An enzyme replacer, available as powder, tablet or capsule, should be added to the food in accordance with the manufacturer's directions.

- Response to the above should be fairly rapid and within 3–5 days the diarrhoea should have ceased, with the animal starting to pass near normal stools. If diarrhoea continues, further investigation may be necessary.

  Once diarrhoea has ceased, the amount of food and enzyme replacer fed should be gradually increased to encourage weight gain. The aim is for a slow steady increase in weight; feeding large amounts of extra food to increase the rate of weight gain will often result in the reappearance of diarrhoea.

- Once the animal has reached its ideal body weight, the amount fed may be reduced to a maintenance level. At this point the amount of enzyme replacer used should also be reduced to the lowest amount necessary to maintain weight and normal faeces. If the animal continues on the low-fat, highly digestible diet without any additions, only a minimum amount of enzyme replacer is necessary.

- Consistency in the type of food, the amount fed and the timing of meals is essential for correct management of EPI.

Steatorrhoea

Streatorrhoea, excess fat in the faeces, is often associated with EPI, although it can occur with other disorders of the intestinal mucosa. Malabsorption of fat in the diet allows it to pass through the intestines and as a consequence the faeces are greasy. They are also bulky, pale in colour and malodorous. Dietary modification, when the cause is other than EPI, includes the use of low to moderate levels of highly digestible fat in a diet appropriate to the underlying disorder.

THE LIVER

The liver is the largest organ in the body. It has a large functional reserve and signs of liver failure do not occur until less than 30% of its functional capacity is left. It is, however, capable of regeneration, provided that a good blood supply is maintained and an adequate level of nutrients is supplied (Figure 7.3).

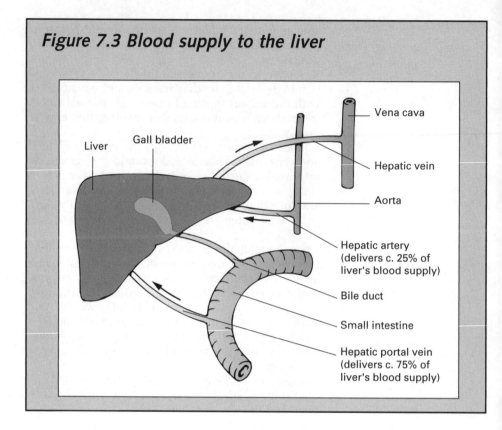

Figure 7.3 Blood supply to the liver

Liver · Gall bladder · Vena cava · Hepatic vein · Aorta · Hepatic artery (delivers c. 25% of liver's blood supply) · Bile duct · Small intestine · Hepatic portal vein (delivers c. 75% of liver's blood supply)

The liver is involved in metabolism of all nutrients and the storage of several, particularly glycogen, iron and vitamins A and D (Figure 7.4). It is responsible for the production and excretion of bile, the synthesis of clotting factors and is also the body's 'detox' unit. Compounds which enter the body through the gut are passed along the hepatic portal vein to the liver where toxic products are removed. These are then excreted either via the kidneys in urine or in the bile. With this wide range of biochemical functions, it is clear that any disruption in normal functioning of the liver will have far-reaching effects.

There are several causes of liver malfunction including infection, toxins, trauma and neoplasms, while metabolic disorders interfere with normal activities. A physical abnormality, portosystemic shunt, carries blood directly into the systemic circulation, bypassing the liver. This effectively deprives the animal of nutrients because normal metabolism is not possible and also 'poisons' it, because circulating toxins and waste products are not removed and excreted. Portosystemic shunts may be congenital (seen especially in Yorkshire Terriers) or acquired. Surgical correction is sometimes possible.

Figure 7.4 Nutrient metabolism in the liver

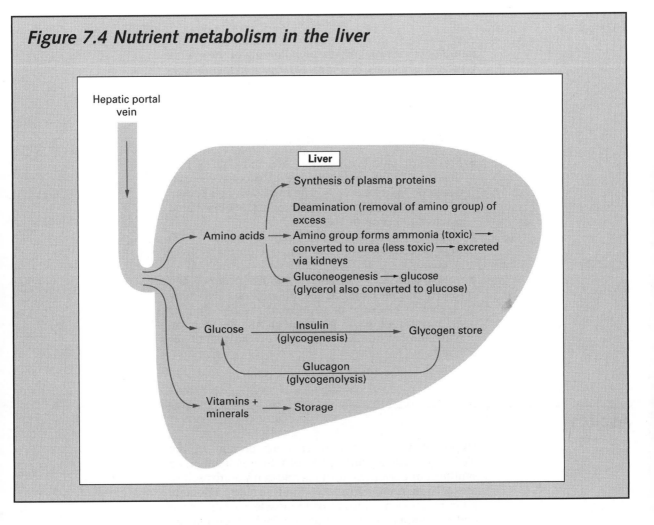

Congenital portosystemic shunts produce clinical signs in young animals. They are often stunted and advanced cases may develop hepatic encephalopathy. (Hepatic encephalopathy may also develop in older animals with cirrhosis, when fibrous tissue replaces normal parenchymal tissue.) This form of brain degeneration is thought to be due to the accumulation of toxic products which arise from bacterial breakdown of nutrients in the gastrointestinal tract, in particular ammonia. Since ammonia is also a waste product of protein metabolism, animals suffering from hepatic encephalopathy may need to be fed a diet that is very low in protein. This is contrary to the usual dietary recommendation of a moderate level of protein to counteract impaired protein synthesis and enable the liver to regenerate whenever possible.

Two clinical signs often associated with, but not exclusive to, liver disease are jaundice and ascites.

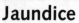

Jaundice

Jaundice (or icterus) produces yellowing of the sclerae (where it is usually first noticed), mucous membranes and skin. This yellowing is due to abnormally high levels of bilirubin, a breakdown product of haemoglobin, which is normally conjugated in the liver and excreted in bile. There are three types of jaundice, only one of which is directly related to liver disease:

- Prehepatic jaundice occurs when bilirubin is produced in large quantities due to excessive breakdown of red blood cells. The excessive breakdown of red blood cells may be due to immune-mediated disease, infection or toxins.
- Hepatic (or hepatocellular) jaundice results from impaired liver function due to primary liver disease.
- Post-hepatic (or obstructive) jaundice occurs when bile is unable to reach the duodenum. This may be due to blockage or rupture of the bile duct or as a result of some blockage in the duodenum. Nutrition has no direct influence on the quantity of bile.

Ascites

Hypoproteinaemia, a deficiency of protein in the blood, has several causes, one of which is inadequate synthesis of protein in the liver, and can lead to ascites, the accumulation of serous fluid in the abdomen. Hypoproteinaemia also leads to muscle wastage as the body attempts to compensate for lack of protein by using muscle protein. In these cases the animal's protein requirement may be higher than normal to compensate both for poor absorption and synthesis and to allow for hepatic regeneration.

Ascites can also be affected by the sodium content of the diet and its influence on water retention by the kidneys. Moderate sodium restriction is recommended for animals with liver disease.

Glucose intolerance

The liver plays an important role in the regulation of blood glucose levels and disruption of this function may result in glucose intolerance, an inability to absorb and utilize glucose. Insulin becomes less effective and is therefore required in larger quantities; this in turn places extra strain on the endocrine pancreas.

It is clear then that liver disease is not a single entity but a series of malfunctions and diseases, each of which will have different effects on the body. There is no one diet that is ideal for use in all liver conditions. That said, given the complexities of liver functions and liver diseases, it would be very difficult to design individual diets for each affected animal. Proprietary diets are available that address the major necessities and these are usually the best option in dietary management.

Whenever possible the underlying cause should be identified and treated but dietary management is very important. Anorexia and malnutrition compounded by anorexia are common in animals with liver disorders and nutritional support is essential.

Dietary modification aims to:

- meet the animal's basic needs for nutrients
- support regeneration of damaged tissue
- slow progression of the disease and ameliorate existing signs
- prevent further complications.

This is achieved by providing:

- a palatable diet
- an energy-dense diet with moderate levels of fat (with the correct $n-6$ to $n-3$ ratio) and digestible complex carbohydrates, e.g. rice
- moderate amounts of high-quality protein, e.g. cottage cheese and egg
- increased levels of water-soluble vitamins, especially B complex vitamins
- increased levels of vitamin K if there are coagulation problems. Liver patients are often deficient in vitamin E, but it is important not to over-supplement this vitamin
- moderately decreased levels of sodium to reduce water retention
- increased levels of zinc, commonly deficient in animals with liver disease.

As always when the digestive system is compromised, small meals fed often is the rule.

Copper storage disease

Copper storage disease is a largely inherited disorder which occurs in a high percentage of Bedlington Terriers (and crosses with this breed). Damage to hepatic tissue occurs when copper levels in the liver rise due to impaired removal.

Affected animals require a diet low in copper, and zinc supplementation may be helpful as zinc and copper compete for the same absorption sites, zinc being absorbed in preference to copper. The damage is irreversible so it has been suggested that susceptible animals should be fed a low-copper diet as early as possible and continue on this diet throughout their lives. Foods that are likely to be high in copper, e.g. liver and mineral supplements, should be avoided.

Hepatic lipidosis

Hepatic lipidosis is a disease characterized by an accumulation of triglycerides in the liver to a point beyond that considered normal. The liver may be damaged by the physical presence of these high levels of fat or by hepatotoxic agents to which it becomes more susceptible in the presence of excess fat.

Feline hepatic lipidosis is commonest in obese cats that have not eaten for several days. Liver function is impaired and the prognosis is often poor. This disease is common in North America but not elsewhere, which may be related to the high percentage of obese cats in that country. As the proportion of overweight cats increases in other countries, it is possible that hepatic lipidosis will become more common. For this reason it is important that dieting cats should be force fed if not eating voluntarily within 3 days.

Recovery from feline hepatic lipidosis takes several weeks, requiring constant nutritional support, and the use of indwelling feeding tubes should be considered.

REPRODUCTIVE DISEASE

Some problems that occur in the dam during pregnancy and lactation can be related to inadequate nutrition both before and after conception of the young. Poor nutrition contributes, among other things, to low conception rates, fetal abnormalities and poor milk production.

Animals that are not in peak condition at the time of mating will have inadequate body stores of nutrients and energy to sustain the growing fetuses and will end the pregnancy in poor condition, particularly when poor-quality diets with low digestibility continue to be fed through this period.

Persistent diarrhoea may occur when the dam attempts to satisfy the increasing energy demands on her body by eating more. A poor quality diet will lead to excessive intake which further reduces digestibility and the overwhelmed gut is unable to cope with the quantity of food ingested. Diarrhoea results and damages the gut, exacerbating the problem. Without some dietary improvement, the bitch or queen is on a downward spiral, with detrimental effects on both dam and fetal development.

Inadequate nutrition often results in anaemia in both dam and neonates and may be a factor in the 'fading puppy (or kitten) syndrome'. Lactation will also be affected: inadequate amounts of colostrum and milk will be produced, reducing the growth rates and viability of the neonates.

Most of these problems will be avoided if the dam receives adequate nutrition as outlined in the lifestage section.

Eclampsia

Eclampsia, otherwise known as puerperal tetany, is caused by falling plasma levels of calcium (and often also magnesium) and a failure of the body to compensate for the calcium lost in the milk. This is usually linked to inadequate diet.

Eclampsia can occur in both bitches and queens but most frequently affects bitches with large litters and is more common in small breeds. It usually occurs 3–4 weeks after giving birth, i.e. at the time of peak demand for milk from the pups. Symptoms will vary from restlessness and panting in mild cases, through muscle tremors to convulsions in the most severe cases. Treatment is with calcium supplementation. In mild cases this can be given orally but when the symptoms are more severe, intravenous administration will be required. Yet again prevention is better than cure and feeding an energy-dense growth diet ad lib during lactation, will lessen the chances of eclampsia occurring.

Pups should be encouraged to take solid food from the age of 3 weeks, particularly when the litter is large, to decrease the demand for milk.

THE URINARY SYSTEM

The urinary tract, as a major excretory system for the body, is affected by the diet in a variety of ways. Like the liver, the kidneys have a large functional reserve and also like the liver, signs of renal failure do not appear until approximately 70% of functional tissue is lost. Unlike the liver, the kidneys do not regenerate, so measures that slow progression of renal disease are very important. In some cases surviving nephrons will enlarge (hypertrophy) to compensate for lack of

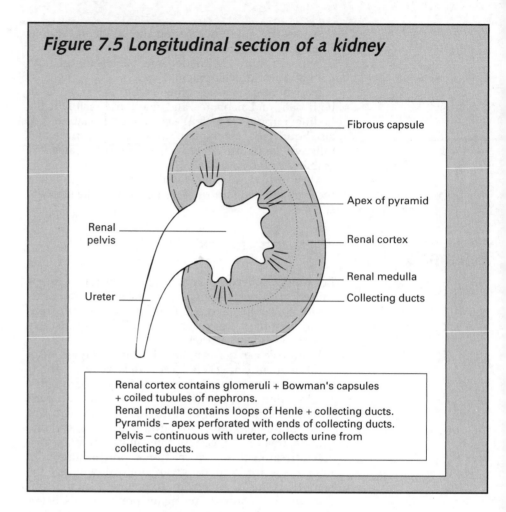

Figure 7.5 Longitudinal section of a kidney

Fibrous capsule

Renal pelvis

Apex of pyramid

Renal cortex

Renal medulla

Collecting ducts

Ureter

Renal cortex contains glomeruli + Bowman's capsules + coiled tubules of nephrons.
Renal medulla contains loops of Henle + collecting ducts.
Pyramids – apex perforated with ends of collecting ducts.
Pelvis – continuous with ureter, collects urine from collecting ducts.

numbers and the animal enters a state known as 'compensated renal disease' when kidney function appears to have returned to normal. Unfortunately, this compensation is limited and the extra stress on the surviving nephrons leads to further deterioration of the kidneys. Clinical signs reappear and renal failure develops.

Kidneys (Figure 7.5) work on the 'sieve and recycle' basis – waste products are eliminated from the body and useful products resorbed (Figure 7.6). When normal function is disrupted, toxic products of protein breakdown remain in the circulation causing azotaemia and products normally retained are lost.

The urinary tract is also the major system regulating the fluid needs of the body. Water is resorbed in the kidney tubule, concentrating the urine and maintaining fluid balance within the body. Excess water is excreted. The ability to concentrate urine decreases as functional loss increases, and polyuria with con-

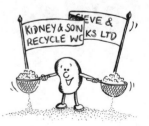

Figure 7.6 A single nephron (filtration unit)

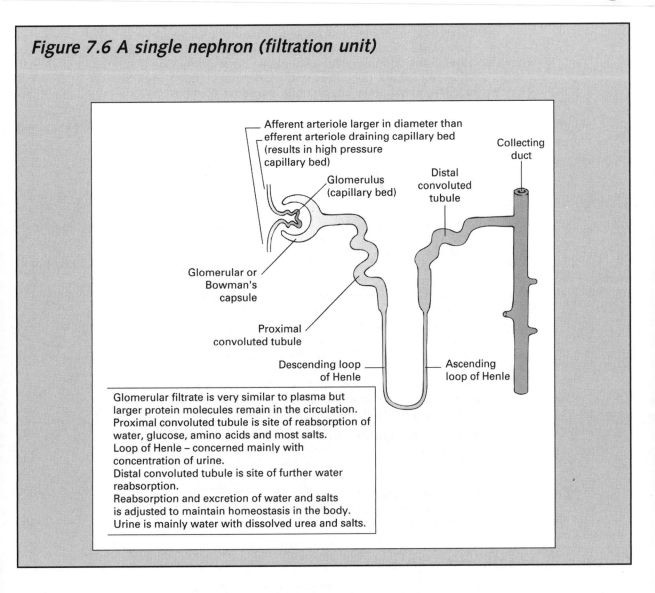

Afferent arteriole larger in diameter than efferent arteriole draining capillary bed (results in high pressure capillary bed)

Glomerulus (capillary bed)

Distal convoluted tubule

Collecting duct

Glomerular or Bowman's capsule

Proximal convoluted tubule

Descending loop of Henle

Ascending loop of Henle

Glomerular filtrate is very similar to plasma but larger protein molecules remain in the circulation.
Proximal convoluted tubule is site of reabsorption of water, glucose, amino acids and most salts.
Loop of Henle – concerned mainly with concentration of urine.
Distal convoluted tubule is site of further water reabsorption.
Reabsorption and excretion of water and salts is adjusted to maintain homeostasis in the body.
Urine is mainly water with dissolved urea and salts.

sequent polydipsia is one of the first signs of chronic renal failure. Polydipsia and polyuria are not, however, exclusive to renal failure and when reported usually require further investigation. Cat owners are much less likely than dog owners to notice these signs in their pets, so renal disease may be more advanced in cats before owners become aware of problems.

Renal failure may be acute or chronic.

Acute renal failure

Acute renal failure is the sudden onset of kidney malfunction due to infection or nephrotoxins which damage the nephrons and cause retention of nitrogenous waste products within the circulation. Factors outside the kidneys can also cause acute kidney failure, e.g. shock (a sudden reduction in renal blood supply), dehydration, trauma (e.g. ruptured bladder) or obstruction (e.g. urolithiasis). These factors are referred to as either pre- or post-renal factors. Physical problems require rapid remedial action to prevent further renal damage. When treated promptly, acute renal failure can be reversed, but untreated it may develop into chronic renal failure.

Management of acute kidney failure

Intravenous fluid therapy will usually be required to correct dehydration and restore electrolyte balance. Fluid therapy also increases perfusion of the kidneys and will help limit or prevent further damage occurring. Care must be taken to avoid fluid overload.

Nutritional support forms an essential aspect of treatment. Animals with acute renal failure are in a catabolic state and have a high turnover of protein. When this protein is used for energy, nitrogenous wastes are produced which exacerbate the existing uraemia and the main consideration should be the provision of adequate energy from non-protein sources to reduce uraemia and encourage renal recovery.

Dietary modification aims to provide:

- calories from highly digestible carbohydrate or fat
- palatability – patients with renal failure are often anorexic and nasogastric tubes may need to be used
- moderate levels of high-quality protein to encourage renal recovery while limiting nitrogenous wastes
- low phosphate levels to limit renal damage.

Chronic renal failure

Chronic renal failure (CRF) is a long-term deterioration of kidney function. This degeneration is part of the normal ageing process and is one of the major causes of non-accidental death in both dogs and cats. Not surprisingly, although it can occur in dogs and cats at any age, it is usually seen as a disease of older animals. It is progressive, the loss of functional reserve being followed by renal insufficiency, at which point clinical signs start to appear as the kidneys are no longer able to function efficiently.

Any of the factors which give rise to acute kidney failure may also contribute to chronic renal failure but, in addition, immunological or congenital disorders or neoplasms may accelerate the natural degeneration of nephrons. The diet plays an important role in the management of CRF .

Dietary modification aims to:

- reduce clinical signs
- minimize mineral and electrolyte imbalances
- slow progression of the disease
- supply energy and nutrient levels that normalize and maintain ideal bodyweight.

This is achieved by providing:

- moderate levels of high-quality protein to reduce nitrogenous wastes but supply sufficient protein for maintenance. Cats will require higher levels than dogs. As CRF progresses, protein restriction may be necessary to control uraemia
- restriction of phosphorus to slow the progression of renal failure
- energy from fat and carbohydrate. Fat provides energy density and increases palatability. The addition of n−3 fatty acids may be advantageous because of their anti-inflammatory properties
- moderate restriction of sodium to reduce or prevent hypertension
- increased levels of water-soluble vitamins to compensate for losses in urine when polyuria is present
- fermentable fibre to encourage increase of bacteria in the large intestine. These use nitrogen in the blood urea for the synthesis of bacterial protein which is then excreted in the faeces
- restriction or supplementation of potassium levels as appropriate. Either hyperkalaemia or hypokalaemia may occur in animals with CRF. Hypokalaemia is the commonest electrolyte imbalance in cats with CRF.

As always in stressed animals, feed little and often. Canned food may be preferable in cats at least, as it encourages water intake and is more palatable than dry foods.

Renal secondary hyperparathyroidism

The amount of phosphorus excreted by diseased kidneys is reduced leading to hyperphosphataemia. This causes an imbalance in the calcium to phosphorus ratio, stimulates release of parathyroid hormone and ultimately leads to demineralization of bone. The mandible is the most noticeably affected bone (this condition is sometimes called 'rubber jaw'). Parathyroid hormone is itself nephrotoxic, so increased levels further damage the kidneys and hyperphosphataemia stimulates calcification of soft tissue. Calcium deposited in the kidney also causes kidney damage.

Calcium levels in the diet may require supplementation, but each case must be assessed and treated individually as wide variations occur in blood calcium levels.

Lower urinary tract disease

Lower urinary tract disease is a term used to describe a variety of conditions including inflammation and infection (cystitis and urethritis) and the formation of calculi (uroliths). Animals suffering from these disorders usually exhibit pain or discomfort when urinating and produce urine that contains varying amounts of blood. They will usually pass urine more frequently and in smaller amounts.

Cystitis

Cystitis, inflammation of the bladder, may be due to external infection but may also result from a physical condition, e.g. urinary retention or the presence of calculi in the bladder. The bladder is lined with a protective layer of epithelial cells and glycosaminoglycan. When this layer is thinner than normal, the bladder is more susceptible to damage and cystitis more likely. Dietary supplements are now available containing glycosaminoglycan which claim to increase this protective layer and to reduce the occurrence of cystitis.

Calculi (uroliths)

Calculi are mineral salts deposited in a protein matrix which form in the hollow organs of the animal's body. Those which form in the urine or in the urinary tract are known as uroliths. They are hard, irritant and increase in size when conditions are favourable.

These calculi may be washed out of the bladder when the animal urinates and if of sufficient size, may block the urethra with potentially fatal consequences. The urethra may also be blocked by 'plugs' consisting of proteins, cell debris and crystals. Male dogs and cats are more prone to urethral plugs than the female of the species because of the length and comparative narrowness of the urethra.

Several conditions have to be met for calculi to form and grow. Controlling any of these conditions will lessen or prevent their formation:

- the mineral must be present in sufficient quantities
- the urine pH must be favourable for precipitation of the mineral
- the crystals must be retained in the bladder for a period long enough to allow formation of the calculi.

Diet plays an important role in the formation of urinary calculi, as the mineral components are acquired through the diet and digestive processes. The pH of the urine and the volume of urine are also affected by diet. Generally speaking, the urine of carnivores is acidic and that of herbivores is alkaline. Feeding large amounts of plant-based foods may change the normal acidic urine of the dog towards a more alkaline one.

Foods which contain a higher than average level of salt will encourage diuresis, and highly digestible foods which leave little residue will decrease the amount of faeces passed and consequently decrease the amount of faecal water. This in turn increases the amount excreted through the kidneys.

In some cases cystitis and the formation of calculi may be linked. If the infection is due to urease-producing bacteria, the level of urea in the urine increases and the likelihood of struvite uroliths forming is increased. These cases require antibiotic therapy in addition to a calculolytic (dissolution) diet. The antibiotics should be continued throughout the period of dissolution as bacteria may be trapped within the urolith. Infection-induced uroliths are more common in dogs than in cats.

Excess weight and inactivity contribute to urolith formation as these animals tend to urinate less often and retained urine allows time for the relevant minerals and salts to be precipitated out. Animals that are confined for long periods, e.g. dogs whose owners are out most of the day, also have this problem of retained urine.

Many cats only drink small amounts and will, as a consequence, have urine with a higher concentration than normal of minerals. These cats are probably best fed a moist food, as the total of water thus consumed is higher than the extra water drunk by cats fed a dry food.

Neutered animals seem to be at increased risk of developing uroliths, possibly because they are more likely to be overweight and less active than entire ones.

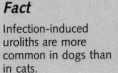

Fact

Infection-induced uroliths are more common in dogs than in cats.

Uroliths

There are several types of urolith which occur in dogs and cats. They are formed under different conditions and require different treatments. These are summarized in Table 7.3. Dietary management also varies for each type.

Table 7.3 **Summary of urolith formation and treatment**

Urolith	Forms in	Treatment
Struvite	Alkaline urine	Calculolytic diet or surgical removal
Calcium oxalate	Variable but usually acidic urine	Surgical removal
Ammonium urate	Acidic urine	Calculolytic diet and allopurinol
Cystine	Acidic urine	Calculolytic diet or surgical removal
Silicate	Usually acidic urine	Surgical removal

Struvite uroliths

Struvite (magnesium-ammonium-phosphate hexahydrate) was originally the most common type of urolith in both dogs and cats but its incidence has decreased in recent years.

Predisposing factors are:

- infection with urease-producing bacteria
- excess magnesium and protein in the diet
- excess calcium which affects the calcium to phosphorus ratio.

The amount of magnesium in proprietary cat foods, particularly dry diets, was a source of concern in the past. As a result, many owners will still be reluctant to feed dry foods to cats and may need reassurance that the problem has been addressed. Proprietary cat foods now contain less magnesium and are designed to promote an acidic urine (but bear in mind that, as stated earlier, those cats with low intake of water may well benefit from being fed moist as opposed to dry foods).

Treatment
Dissolution by dietary modification is the chief method of treatment for these uroliths but surgical removal may be recommended under certain circumstances (see below).

Dietary modification aims to:

- dissolve uroliths present in the bladder
- prevent formation of new uroliths.

This is achieved by providing:

- very low levels of high biological value protein
- reduced amounts of calcium, phosphorus and magnesium

- increased sodium levels
- acidic urine.

The daily amount of this diet should be split into two or three equal portions and should be fed until 3–4 weeks after the uroliths are no longer visible radiographically. Just as blood glucose levels increase after a meal, so the pH of urine increases after eating, the 'post-prandial alkaline tide'; the more food eaten, the higher the pH. Feeding smaller amounts more often, levels out the pH fluctuations and reduces the risk of struvite formation.

In some animals this calculolytic diet is inappropriate. It should not be fed to pregnant or lactating animals or those suffering from congestive heart failure, renal or hepatic disease. In these animals the uroliths should be surgically removed. Feeding this calculolytic diet to growing animals may result in stunted growth because of low protein levels. In these cases, the diet should be fed with care and only until the uroliths are no longer radiographically visible.

Calcium oxalate uroliths

These are the second most common urolith in dogs and cats and are now seen with increased frequency.
Predisposing factors are:

- diets high in calcium (especially dairy products), sodium (increases calcium excretion) and oxalates (plants and vegetables)
- supplements of vitamin D (increased absorption of calcium from the diet) and vitamin C (oxalic acid is a metabolite of ascorbic acid)
- age – calcium oxalate crystals appear more frequently in older animals, particularly older cats.

Treatment
There is as yet no calculolytic diet available for calcium oxalate uroliths so surgical removal is recommended. Attention should be paid to those predisposing factors which can be influenced by diet in susceptible animals.

Ammonium urate uroliths

These are seen infrequently in dogs and cats.
Predisposing factors are:

- high-protein diets, particularly those containing muscle or organ tissue. Muscle and organ tissues have large numbers of cells and therefore cell nuclei. Urates (salts of uric acid) are metabolites of purines which occur in DNA and RNA

- liver dysfunction, in particular portosystemic shunts
- gender – males are more susceptible than females to the formation of these uroliths
- breed – Dalmatians are particularly susceptible as they lack uricase, an enzyme which converts uric acid to allantoin. These dogs therefore excrete more urates than other breeds.

Treatment
These uroliths are often surgically removed but calculolytic diets are possible.
  Dietary modification aims to provide:

- reduced levels of protein, in particular nucleic acids. Milk protein (casein) and eggs are suitable protein sources
- increased levels of non-protein calories
- supplements of allopurinol which inhibits production of uric acid
- alkaline urine.

Like the calculolytic diet for struvite, this diet should be fed until 3–4 weeks after the uroliths are no longer radiographically visible. Ammonium urate uroliths are not always radiodense and contrast radiography may be necessary to highlight them.
  These diets are contraindicated for very young animals and pregnant or lactating females.

Cystine uroliths

These occur infrequently in dogs and only very rarely in cats. They are caused by an inherited metabolic defect chiefly occurring in male dogs. Dissolution of cystine uroliths may be achieved with a diet similar to that designed for dissolution of ammonium urate uroliths (supplements of allopurinol are not required) but surgical removal is more often recommended.

Silicate uroliths

These occur only in dogs and most often in males, particularly German Shepherds.
  Predisposing factors are:

- eating soil
- diets high in plant proteins.

Treatment
Surgical removal is usually recommended.

Failure of calculolytic diets

When uroliths fail to dissolve despite feeding a calculolytic diet, the following questions should be asked:

- is the urolith of mixed composition?
- was the diagnosis of urolith type correct?
- is the diet being fed correctly?
- are other foods being given?

Recurrence of uroliths

Many animals that form stones will form them again unless preventative measures are taken. Prevention and owner compliance are particularly important when genetic or metabolic functions are involved, as the predisposing factors cannot be removed. Prevention is also important in those cases where surgical removal is the best or only option, as repeated surgery is undesirable.

Struvite uroliths

Since the dissolution diet for these is very low in protein, it is not appropriate for long-term use. Diets which prevent recurrence have a higher protein level (but still lower than normal maintenance diets) and normal sodium levels. Calories should be provided from non-protein sources. The diet should ensure that urine remains acidic.

Calcium oxalate, ammonium urate and cystine uroliths

Preventative diets for these are the same as those for dissolution of urate and cystine uroliths. These diets are suitable for long-term maintenance in adults but are relatively low in protein so the animal should be monitored for protein malnutrition. Adequate calories should be supplied from a non-protein source.

Silicate uroliths

The ingestion of soil should be prevented and protein provided from an animal source.

THE ENDOCRINE SYSTEM

Diabetes mellitus and hyper/hypothyroidism are the most common endocrine disorders seen in the dog and cat. Cushing's disease and Addison's disease are also endocrine disorders but are seen less frequently. The effect of diet on diabetes mellitus has been studied for some time and dietary management nowadays goes hand in hand with drug therapy, but dietary recommendations for other endocrine disorders are scanty.

Diabetes mellitus

Glucose is the main biological fuel of the body's cells and its concentration in the blood is carefully regulated to ensure that all tissues are supplied according to their need. Regulation (Figure 7.7) is achieved by two sets of opposing hormones; several hormones are responsible for raising blood glucose levels but insulin, produced by the endocrine pancreas, is the only major hormone involved in lowering levels. Consequently a lack of insulin or a decrease in its efficiency allows the actions of the blood glucose raising hormones to continue unopposed, upsetting the normal balance and having a profound effect on the body.

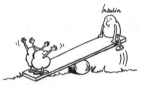

Too many blood glucose raising hormones upset the normal balance

Insulin also has a role to play in protein and fat metabolism and disruption will occur in both of these processes when insulin is lacking. The breakdown of fat deposits to fatty acids and ketones may lead to the development of ketoacidosis which is potentially fatal.

A deficiency of insulin may be due either to a reduction in the amount released by the pancreas (decreased production, or absence or destruction of insulin-producing islet cells) or an increase in levels of opposing hormones. Transient diabetes mellitus can occur in entire bitches during that part of the oestrus cycle when progesterone levels are high, progesterone being one of the hormones responsible for increasing blood glucose levels (Figure 7.8).

The efficiency of insulin may be reduced in overweight animals when the insulin receptor sites become 'hidden' by fat layers. Loss of weight in these animals will uncover some of these 'hidden' sites, allowing the circulating insulin to become more effective and reversing the signs of diabetes mellitus. If however the animal has been overweight for some time, loss of weight may not produce this reversal, as when receptor sites are hidden the body is encouraged to produce extra insulin to compensate, which can lead to exhaustion of the islet cells.

Humans suffering from diabetes mellitus are treated either with tablets, hypoglycaemic drugs, which encourage increases in both production and efficiency

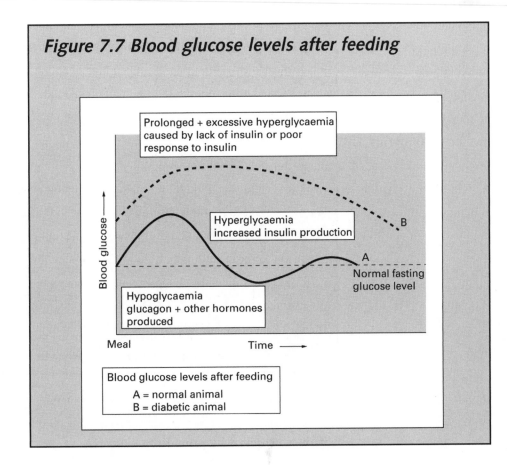

Figure 7.7 Blood glucose levels after feeding

Prolonged + excessive hyperglycaemia caused by lack of insulin or poor response to insulin

Hyperglycaemia increased insulin production

B

A

Normal fasting glucose level

Hypoglycaemia glucagon + other hormones produced

Blood glucose

Meal

Time

Blood glucose levels after feeding
A = normal animal
B = diabetic animal

of insulin, or with insulin injections. Their diet will also be carefully controlled.

Hypoglycaemic drugs may be used in a small percentage of cats with diabetes mellitus but are generally thought to be of little value in the treatment of affected dogs. Dietary modification is always required and in cats this change of diet may be sufficient to control the symptoms. Treatment of diabetes mellitus requires regularity and consistency in the administering of drugs, exercise and feeding.

Dietary modification aims to:

- minimize post-mealtime (post-prandial) fluctuations in blood glucose levels
- maximize the efficiency of endogenous and administered insulin
- provide the optimum amounts of nutrients with a calorie density designed to maintain an ideal body weight. Obese animals will require less calories; underweight animals will initially require extra calories.

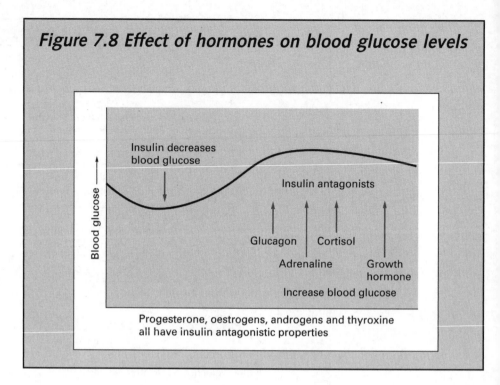

Figure 7.8 Effect of hormones on blood glucose levels

Blood glucose

Insulin decreases blood glucose

Insulin antagonists

Glucagon   Cortisol

Adrenaline   Growth hormone

Increase blood glucose

Progesterone, oestrogens, androgens and thyroxine all have insulin antagonistic properties

This is achieved by providing:

- a fixed formula food to ensure consistency
- a diet low in simple sugars and high in complex carbohydrates to slow glucose absorption
- reduced fat content to lower blood lipid levels
- a diet high in fibre, with a mix of both soluble and insoluble forms. These slow absorption of glucose and reduce fluctuations in blood glucose levels. Soluble fibre helps to reduce total lipid and triglyceride content of the liver and helps prevent rises in serum lipid levels
- moderate levels of high biological value protein to ensure adequate, but not excessive, supplies of amino acids.

The recommended levels in man are:

Complex carbohydrate	60%
Protein	20%
Fat	20%.

These are also thought to be effective levels for the dietary management of diabetes in dogs. Cats will require higher protein and lower carbohydrate levels.

Although high-fibre diets are recommended as an aid to controlling blood glucose levels, their introduction can cause problems. They can cause constipation if not introduced gradually and, as they tend to be less palatable, they may not be accepted by all animals. They are usually low in calories and so should not be fed to thin diabetic animals until they have regained weight.

Changing to a high-fibre diet shortly after diagnosis is often helpful but in other cases, when the animal is reluctant to eat the new diet, stabilization can be difficult and it may be necessary to continue on the animal's normal diet at this stage. Dietary changes can be attempted again once the animal is stable and insulin doses adjusted accordingly.

The amount of water drunk is a good indication of the level of diabetic control and owners should monitor this daily.

Semi-moist foods are often preserved by the addition of glucose, so should not be fed to diabetic animals.

Feeding regimes

Feeding regimes are very important but they must be acceptable to the animal and practical for the owner if they are to be adhered to. When diabetic control is by diet alone, small meals several times daily will reduce post-prandial blood glucose fluctuations and reduce the amount of nutrients absorbed at any one time.

When injections of insulin are given, meal times should coincide with maximum insulin activity. The length of time between injection and maximum insulin activity will vary between individuals and part of the stabilization process is to determine this period.

The majority of diabetic patients will receive one injection per day. This is most often given in the morning but the owner's lifestyle may indicate another, better time for this to be administered. It is usual for one-third of the day's total ration to be fed at the time of injection and the remaining two-thirds given 8–10 hours later to coincide with peak insulin activity.

Some animals will require two injections of insulin daily. In these cases the daily ration should ideally split into four equal portions, two being given at the time of the injections and two midway between injections. If this is not practical, the daily ration may be fed in two equal portions at the times of insulin administration. Cats may be reluctant to eat at prescribed meal times and, in these cases, continual access to food should be allowed (although the amount provided should be measured and should not exceed the daily ration).

It is important to remind owners that having established a routine they should stick to it as much as possible – weekend variations are not encouraged. Maintaining a routine is particularly difficult for shift workers and at holiday times but it is in the animal's best interests to minimize disruptions – a diabetic's life can be unadventurous and boring.

Cushing's disease (hyperadrenocorticism)

This is caused by overproduction of the adrenal cortex hormones and occurs chiefly in older dogs and cats due to pituitary tumour or neoplasia in the adrenal glands themselves. It can also be induced by over-administration of corticosteroid drugs.

The hormones produced are antagonistic to insulin and may give rise to hyperglycaemia. Dietary recommendations for these animals are therefore similar to those for diabetic animals.

Addison's disease (hypoadrenocorticism)

This is caused by a lack of the hormones produced by the adrenal cortex. Clinical signs are normally only seen in the dog. It is treated medically and there are no specific dietary recommendations. These dogs do seem however to benefit from a regular routine with smaller, more frequent meals and, like diabetics, do best when exercise levels are moderate and without daily variation.

Hyperthyroidism and hypothyroidism

Both of these conditions involve malfunction of the thyroid gland. Hyperthyroidism is commonest in cats and hypothyroidism commonest in dogs.

Excess thyroid production in the cat often results in loss of weight. These cats are usually in the age group classed as geriatric and some will be very elderly. Often the cat has other concurrent illness, e.g. chronic renal failure.

Dietary modification aims to:

● increase calorie content to restore lost weight

- provide protein and fat levels appropriate to geriatric cats
- consider dietary requirements for other, concurrent illness.

Reduced thyroid levels in the dog will give rise to a variety of clinical signs, including weight gain. The condition is likely to be treated medically and there are no specific dietary recommendations, although calorie restriction may be considered for some overweight dogs.

Hyperlipidaemia

Animals with hyperlipidaemia have a high lipid concentration in their blood while they are fasting. The condition may occur secondary to endocrine or metabolic disorders or as a primary disease resulting from an inherited disorder.

When it occurs secondary to another condition, treatment of the underlying disorder will usually correct hyperlipidaemia. In other cases dietary modification is recommended to alleviate clinical signs.

Dietary modification aims to:

- reduce fat content to lower blood lipid levels
- provide calorie density at a level which prevents long-term weight loss but avoids excess energy input
- provide increased fibre levels to reduce lipid absorption from the gut.

Suitable proprietary diets are to be preferred, as the fat content of home-made diets is likely to vary from day to day.

Questions

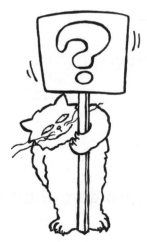

Obesity

1. The normal adult dog has around ___ body fat. _____ normally have a higher body fat content than _____.
2. Commercial reducing diets all have _ _____ calorie content while _____ levels of other nutrients.

3. A successful weight loss programme combines _____ in calorie intake with __ _____ in exercise.

Starvation

1. Animals showing evidence of skeletal muscle loss are in urgent need of nutritional support. True or false?
2. What should be done first for the animal suffering from starvation?
3. What is PEM?
4. Tumour tissue relies on glucose as its fuel source. True or false?

Skeletal disease

1. Nutritionally-related skeletal disorders occur only in young animals. True or false?
2. There is a risk that calcium deficiencies may occur when dogs are fed a vegetarian diet. Why?
3. A diet high in _____ but low in _____ may lead to nutritional secondary hyperparathyroidism. This causes _____ in young animals and _____ in adults.
4. Name two dietary supplements available for treatment of joint disease.

Neuromuscular disease

1. Neuromuscular disorders linked to diet are usually concerned with deficiencies of minerals. True or false?
2. The commonest example of a neuromuscular disorder linked to diet is inadequate levels of _____ in the diet leading to a reduction in _____ ____ .
3. Dietary modification aims to _____ _____ and _____ _____ _____ of muscle and nerves.

Disorders of the integument

1. Skin has only a limited range of responses to deficiencies, disease or irritants. True or false?

2. Up to __% of the daily protein requirement is needed for maintenance of ____ and ____ growth. A _____ deficiency of protein may occur at times of peak demand for protein, e.g. late pregnancy and during _____ , or when very ___ protein diets are being fed because of other, unrelated problems.

3. Some skin conditions will respond to dietary supplementation with essential fatty acids. The response may, however, take sometime to become apparent. For how long should owners continue the supplement before a decision can be made as to its effectiveness?

4. Dietary modification aims to reduce symptoms and repair damage by supplying a balanced diet and supplementation when necessary. Supplementation should, however, be used with care. Why?

5. When might an exclusion diet be recommended?

Cardiovascular disease

1. Which amino acid has been associated with dilated cardiomyopathy in cats? Increased levels of this amino acid are also useful for dogs with heart conditions. True or false?

2. The degree of restriction in levels of sodium, chloride and potassium in diets intended for animals suffering from heart disease should be related to the ____ therapy being used.

3. Some animals with a heart condition will be underweight while others may be overweight. The _____ _____ of the diet should therefore, be appropriate to the animal's condition.

Digestive system

1. _____ indicates a problem in the pharynx or oesophagus; _____ indicates a problem in the stomach or small intestines.

2. List the three functions of the gastrointestinal tract directly related to the food ingested.

3. Vomiting may be caused by factors outside the gastrointestinal tract. True or false?

4. Chronic diarrhoea has two main causes. These are ____ and _____. One of the commonest causes of diarrhoea in the dog is _____ (inflammation of the _____).

5. Inflammation of the small intestines has a greater effect on the animal than inflammation of the large intestines. Why?

6. Dietary management of constipation aims to produce a soft but formed stool. Insoluble, poorly fermentable fibre is beneficial because it increases _____ _____ and _____ _____ of the faeces.

7. The pancreas has both _____ and _____ functions. The _____ secretions form the pancreatic juice, which includes _____ _____ to neutralize the gastric contents and _____ to digest carbohydrates, fats and proteins.

8. What does EPI stand for? What term is used to describe the excessively fatty faeces which are often associated with EPI?

9. Pancreatic enzymes are secreted in an inactive form. Why is this?

10. Which physical abnormality carries blood directly from the gut to the systemic circulation, bypassing the liver?

11. Copper storage disease in the liver is a largely inherited disorder. Which breed is most likely to be affected.

12. Jaundice is always indicative of primary liver disease. True or false?

Reproductive system

1. Adequate nutrition of the dam both before and after conception has an important effect on the health of the dam and the viability of the offspring. True or false?

2. Eclampsia occurs most frequently in _____ with large litters. It is more common in _____ breeds and usually occurs at the time of _____ _____.

Urinary system

1. Polydipsia and polyuria are symptoms exclusive to renal failure. True or false?

2. List four causes of acute renal failure.

3. What is the term applied to long-term deterioration of kidney function?

4. Excretion of phosphorus tends to be decreased in diseased kidneys, leading to hyperphosphataemia. What condition can this lead on to?

5. Animals suffering from lower urinary tract disorders usually exhibit _____ or _____ when urinating. They will usually pass urine more _____ and in _____ amounts. This urine often contains _____.

6. All uroliths may be eliminated by the use of calculoloytic diets. True or false?

Endocrine system

1. Give two reasons why a lack of insulin or a decrease in its efficiency has a profound effect on the body.
2. Fibre plays an important role in glycaemic control because it _____ absorption of glucose and reduces _____ in blood glucose levels.
3. Routine is very important for diabetic patients. True or false?
4. What are the aims of dietary modification for a cat suffering from hyperthyroidism?

Small furries

INTRODUCTION

Not so long ago, rabbits and small rodents were classed as exotics but their increasing popularity has given rise to the need for a more appropriate title for this group of pets. For obvious reasons 'small furries' is now the generally accepted term for rabbits and the small rodents kept as pets – chinchillas, chipmunks, gerbils, guinea-pigs, hamsters, mice and rats – and distinguishes them from other species more worthy of the title 'exotic'. In common with true exotics, however, a large percentage of the problems that occur in these animals is related to husbandry and diet.

Having grouped these rodents and rabbits together under one title, it is tempting to think of them as all having the same nutritional requirements, which is not the case. It is important to remember that:

- each species has its own nutritional requirements
- these requirements are often inadequately provided for.

Dogs and cats have been domesticated for thousands of years and throughout that time cats have remained obligate carnivores. Pest control, one of the major roles in the cat–human relationship has of course, encouraged this reliance on meat. We may have changed their attitude to humans but not their need for meat.

During the period of domestication, we have selectively bred dogs for different types of conformation and temperament; breeding dogs for herding, guarding and companionship to name but three roles. In doing so we also selected (sometimes inadvertently) those animals which were best adapted to living with humans and those which did well on the diet that humans were able to provide. Despite this we have changed the dog's nutritional requirements very little. Wild dogs are chiefly carnivores, while domestic dogs, although veering more to the role of omnivore, are still basically carnivores and at times of stress their bodies respond best to a diet based on meat.

It should come as no surprise, then, to find that species that have been domesticated for far shorter periods have the same nutritional requirements as their wild counterparts. To some extent dogs and, in particular, cats have been free to roam and find food for themselves. Small pets are not so fortunate. They are usually kept caged with little or no access to the external environment and are totally dependent on the food supplied by their owners. If they are not to suffer from nutritional inadequacies, this diet should mimic whenever possible the diet of their wild relatives.

Attention also needs to be paid to their natural feeding habits, e.g. nocturnal, arboreal, etc. Although individuals can and will adapt to strange foods, feeding times and places, they will be more willing to eat and their digestive systems will work better if food is provided when and where they are naturally programmed to find it.

In the wild these animals have to work hard and often cover long distances to find sufficient food, so when kept as pets, food supplied 'on tap' leads to overeating and obesity, lack of exercise (which exacerbates the obesity) and boredom – not a recipe for a fit and healthy life.

SELECTIVE FEEDING

Selective feeding has the potential to cause problems in all species (including humans) but particularly in small mammals. When a variety of foods are supplied free choice, an animal will choose to eat first those items that it prefers. When the total quantity of food is larger than the animal needs to satisfy its energy requirements, then some food is left and the animal has consumed an unbalanced diet, even if the original mix was nutritionally balanced. The Victorian nanny who made her charges eat bread and butter before cake, was preventing selective feeding and encouraging the children to eat a balanced diet.

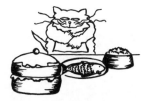

Diet is a matter of choice

Selective feeding is a normal activity and does of course occur in the wild, but there preferences are seasonal or limited by locality, so overall the balance is not unduly disturbed. Owners have access to supplies which override seasons and distance, so that most preferences are available all year round.

One way to prevent selective feeding is to assemble a balanced diet, mix and mill all the ingredients together and produce a pelleted food. All the pellets contain the same proportions of nutrients and the animal therefore consumes a balanced diet. These pellets are commercially produced, so consistency of nutrient composition can be assumed and it is possible for manufacturers to vary the proportions of nutrients to suit different species, or lifestages within a species. Pellets have the added advantage of remaining consistent throughout the bag. Coarse mixes tend to separate out after packing and should be mixed by inverting the bag or box before each feed. Pellets are usually well accepted by the animals but owners often perceive them as boring, adding treats and extras to provide variety. Treats will naturally be those items that the animal prefers and, when fed to excess, the imbalanced diet is back.

A balanced diet formed from a mix of ingredients satisfies the owner's need for variety and meets the animal's needs. It is also closer to the natural diet, takes longer to eat and provides coarser fibre. To ensure that the animal eats a balanced diet it is necessary to read the labels on feeding stuffs carefully. Some coarse mixes are complementary foods and require provision of other dietary components. The newer mixes are more likely to be complete foods.

When buying loose animal feed from the pet shop by weight rather than ready packed, it is not always clearly shown what type of food is on offer, nor are recommended daily quantities readily available. Reputable retailers should be able to supply this information on request.

Mixed ration foods should be fed twice daily, the recommended daily amount being split into two equal portions. Any food left (provided that it is fresh and uncontaminated) is surplus to requirements and the daily ration should be adjusted downwards. This ensures that the whole range of food is eaten. Allowance should be made for the amounts of greenstuffs fed and concentrate rations reduced as necessary. Allowance should also be made for the individual's circumstances. For example, rabbits kept in hutches with little exercise will need less food than is recommended for their size, while those kept outdoors in winter will require extra food to keep them warm during cold spells.

Ad lib feeding is often recommended for young growing pets but this can introduce and encourage selective feeding, a habit which may be difficult to change once they are adult. It is better to feed small amounts often, increasing as necessary, to ensure that a balanced diet is eaten.

RABBITS

The rabbit is now the third most popular pet in Britain, becoming important as a pet for adults which runs contrary to their former image as a children's pet. The veterinary care we are able to provide, and that owners are now willing to pay for, is increasing rapidly and at the centre of this care is the promotion of good nutrition and husbandry.

Rabbits belong to the order of mammals known as Lagomorpha. Lagomorphs are characterized by a second pair of incisors in the upper jaw, compared to the rodents who have a single pair of incisors in both the upper and lower jaws. These extra teeth are small and lie behind the first pair; they are sometimes referred to as the 'peg teeth'.

Rabbits also have more cheek teeth (premolars and molars) than rodents but, in common with rodents, have no canine teeth.

The dental formula is = I2/1, C0/0, P3/2, M3/3.

All the teeth are open-rooted and continue to grow throughout the animal's life.

Although rabbits have lived in Britain since at least the Middle Ages, they originate from Mediterranean countries where their burrowing habits protect them not only from predators but also from cold nights and hot days. Their preferred times of eating, dawn and dusk, reflect this need to avoid the highs and lows of temperature. Even though Britain's climate is more temperate, wild rabbits and many domestic rabbits retain these ancient feeding patterns.

Rabbits are herbivorous selective grazers that in the wild chiefly eat grass. They also eat other green foods including field crops, bark, leaves and some flowers, grain and other seeds, but their chief food is grass. Rabbits will, whenever possible, seek out growing plants, which are richer in protein and soluble carbohydrates than more mature plants but, at the same time, they need to consume reasonably large quantities of insoluble fibre to maintain gut motility.

The fibrous content and the quantities eaten tend to reduce absorption of nutrients and, to counteract this, the rabbit has evolved a complex digestive system, which allows for short transit time but also utilizes as much of the food as possible.

The food is initially thoroughly chewed to break it into smaller particles and mix them with saliva. This mix then passes to the stomach and on into the small intestine where most of the protein, together with some starches and sugars, is absorbed. The residue is then passed along to the junction of the ileum and caecum/colon. Here the rabbit ingeniously separates the remaining ingesta into the non-useful (large particles and indigestible fibre) and the recyclable (small particles and soluble material). The former pass distally through the colon and are excreted as the familiar round, hard droppings.

The portion of ingesta to be recycled passes into the caecum, which in the rabbit is greatly enlarged and is the site of bacterial fermentation of cellulose and other complex carbohydrates. As in other animals, bacterial fermentation results in the production of short-chain fatty acids, which are used as fuel by the cells lining the caecum and can, additionally, be absorbed through the caecal walls into the bloodstream and utilized as an energy source throughout the body. Vitamins are also produced by the bacteria and together with microbial protein are passed back into the colon forming softer, oval droppings known as caecal pellets or caecotrophs. These are coated with mucus as they pass distally through the colon and are then eaten by the rabbit direct from the anus. This is copraphagy or more accurately caecotrophy.

The caecal pellets are swallowed whole and remain in the stomach for several hours. The mucus surrounding them protects them from the acidity of the stomach and allows fermentation to continue. They then pass into the small intestine and are subject to the normal digestive processes. This double passing of food through the body enables the rabbit to obtain more nutrients from the food and utilizes bacteria to supply the extra protein and vitamins not present in sufficient quantities in the basic diet.

It might be expected that increasing the transit time would allow extra nutrients to be absorbed and reduce the need for caecotrophy. Unfortunately, when gut motility is reduced, carbohydrates stay in the intestines longer and encourage the proliferation of bacteria whose preferred substrate is glucose. These bacteria produce enterotoxins with consequent diarrhoea and fluid loss. Without rapid replacement of this fluid, the rabbit is likely to die. Caecotrophy also enables the rabbit to economize on water intake, an asset that enables them to live in more arid conditions than are usually experienced in Britain. It does not, however, exclude the need for provision of fresh, clean water at all times. Rabbits have a daily water requirement roughly equal to 10% of their bodyweight – those fed large quantities of green foods will drink less than those on a dry diet.

Given an adequate supply of grass and hay, water and shelter, rabbits will thrive but, in a domesticated situation, there are many points where this system can break down. Many rabbits are still kept in hutches with (if they are lucky) a run attached; unless the run is moved daily the grass supply is unlikely to be adequate. An increasing number of rabbits are now being kept as house pets and, although this is almost certainly an improvement in comfort, their access to grass may be even more limited. Grass grown out-doors in large seed trays and rotated indoors to supply the house rabbit is one solution, but is unlikely to supply grass in sufficient quantity. Hay is essential for all rabbits and perhaps more so for house rabbits to compensate for the lack of grass. Unfortunately, hay can be messy indoors and owners may be tempted to limit it for this reason. It is better to accept a level of mess in one area and allow the rabbits free access to good-quality hay. Clover hay and alfalfa have a higher level of calcium than grass hay and are useful for young rabbits and pregnant and lactating does, but should not be given to those animals suffering from urolithiasis or those with a very thick urine due to abnormal levels of sediment.

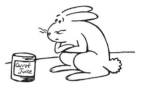

That's not grass!

House rabbits may be tempted to eat house plants, many of which are poisonous (Table 8.1). They also have wider access to human foods and will develop a liking for cake and biscuits if they are given the opportunity.

The difficulty that many owners have in providing adequate quantities of grass and other greenstuffs, together with the misconception still fostered by literature aimed at rabbit owners that rabbits should not be offered greenstuff below the age of 6 months (but see below), has led to the development of several nutritionally-related disorders, the incidence of which seems to be on the increase. Dental problems and obesity are the most common.

Table 8.1 **Poisonous house plants**

All plants grown from bulbs or corms
Aphelandra
Castor oil plant
Diffenbachia
Ferns
Mistletoe
Poinsettia
Umbrella plant

This list is not exhaustive and the best policy is to keep house plants out of reach of house rabbits unless they are known to be non-toxic.

Lifestage feeding

Young rabbits in common with all young animals have a higher requirement for protein and energy per unit of weight than adults. Just as lifestage foods have been developed for dogs and cats, these foods are now becoming available for rabbits, although as yet there are only two stages available, young growing animals and adults. As rabbits continue to increase in popularity and live longer, a closer understanding of their changing requirements may lead to the development of a food for geriatric rabbits.

Young rabbits

Size at maturity varies considerably between the various breeds, from the Netherland Dwarf at 1 kg to the Flemish Giant at 7 kg and over. The majority of rabbits kept as pets are from the small and dwarf breeds and these will generally reach sexual maturity at around 5 months (larger breeds tend to mature later). Up to this stage they require a diet containing 16–18% protein to allow for growth and development, a fat level of around 3% and a fibre content of 16–18%.

Young rabbits will start to be interested in solid food at around 14 days and caecotrophy starts around 3 weeks of age, although they may eat the maternal caecotrophs earlier than this. They are fully weaned at 5–6 weeks.

The food available to the doe determines the type of food the young are introduced to and weaned onto. A doe fed only concentrate rations will have young who are weaned onto concentrates and who have digestive systems with the ability to digest only concentrates. A doe fed concentrates and green foods will have young ones who are weaned onto, and with a digestive system able to cope with, a wider variety of foods. Their delicately balanced digestive system is very sensitive to variations in the diet, so any change should be introduced slowly and carefully. Young rabbits should, whenever possible, be obtained from the breeder and should continue on the same diet for several days before any changes are introduced. This helps to reduce the stress on the rabbit at this stage and helps the transition to its new life. Rabbits obtained from a pet shop or other outlet have probably already had to cope with one change of diet plus the stress of different environments and the challenge of other rabbits in close proximity. In this case it is even more important that the diet provided in the store is fed for the initial week or so in the new home. This is the likely origin of the advice not to feed greens before the age of 6 months.

Adult rabbits

Adults require less protein, around 12–14% is adequate, a fat level of around 1% and at least 20% fibre in their diet, of which half should be insoluble fibre. Regardless of the food the young rabbit is weaned onto, by the time it is adult it should be having greenstuffs and root vegetables which encourage chewing and promote correct wear on the teeth. When the rabbit has access to sufficiently large areas of grazing, concentrate feeding will be unnecessary. All that is required is the provision of clean water and good-quality hay. This is after all the rabbit's natural diet – a fact that many owners overlook.

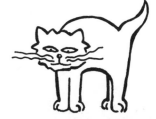

Cautionary notes

Grass should be pulled or cut with scissors or shears, but grass cut by lawnmowers, particularly rotary ones, should not be fed as it can ferment, causing digestive upsets. Grazing grass should not be treated with herbicides and fertilizers are unnecessary (the rabbit does it for you); constant nibbling keeps grass short and sweet. Similarly vegetable and weed plants fed should not have been treated with insecticides.

Very wet foods such as lettuce and fresh spring grass should be fed in small quantities as these can upset the digestive processes and lead to excess gas production, in severe cases causing bloat. Grass which is wet after rain should be fed with care to all rabbits and especially young ones. Food taken from the fridge or frosted grass in winter should similarly be fed with care whatever the age of the rabbit. Rabbits in the wild presumably eat some wet or frosted grass when the need arises, but we do not know how well their digestive systems cope with these products.

> **NB!**
> Grass should be pulled or cut with scissors or shears, but grass cut by lawnmowers, particularly rotary ones, should not be fed as it can ferment, causing digestive upsets.

Table 8.2 Vegetables, fruits and wild plants which may be fed to rabbits (and other small furries)

Vegetables
Beetroot, broccoli, Brussels sprouts, cabbage, carrot, celery, cauliflower, kale, lettuce (small quantities), parsley, radish, spinach, swede, watercress.

Fruits
Apple, blackberry or bramble (and leaves), pear, raspberry (and leaves), strawberry.

Wild plants
Clover, coltsfoot, dandelion, goosegrass, groundsel, milk thistle, raspberry leaves, shepherd's purse, vetches, yarrow

Mixed rations may contain whole, uncrushed peas, beans, maize pips or large pieces of dried locust bean. These have the potential to lodge in the stomach, causing obstruction, and may be fatal. The ration should be checked before feeding and any unmilled items removed.

Table 8.2 lists vegetables, fruits and wild plants that may be offered to rabbits. They should all be fed in moderation and in variety. Shop-bought vegetables will be some time away from being picked and the vitamin content will be degrading, so home-grown are best. New foods should be introduced one by one and any that cause diarrhoea avoided in future. Twigs and small branches from hawthorn and fruit trees can be offered for gnawing exercise.

Breeding stock

Pregnant does require extra protein and energy and a diet similar to that for youngsters is suitable. The amounts fed can be gradually increased and should be offered more frequently, until towards the end of pregnancy ad lib feeding is offered.

Lactating does also require extra food and water, the peak demand being when the young are 2–3 weeks old. After this they will be taking reasonable amounts of solid food and demand for milk will fall.

In the wild, does suckle their young only once or twice daily. Owners new to rabbit breeding may worry that the doe is ignoring her young, but this is normal.

Bran mashes (bran mixed with warm water) used to be recommended for pregnant and lactating does and seem to be enjoyed. Bran is, however, high in phosphorus and low in calcium, so should only be fed in small quantities.

Old age

There are no specific recommendations for dietary care in older rabbits but it is safe to assume that, in common with other animals, their body systems become less efficient with age. Weight and condition changes will offer clues as to how well they are coping; careful observation and weight checks, important throughout life, become even more important now. They may be less able to cope with extremes of temperature and need warmth in winter and cooler conditions in summer. Their food intake may vary too. Possible dental problems may affect what they are able to eat, e.g. carrots previously offered whole may now require slicing or dicing. Each rabbit is an individual and should be treated as such.

Clinical nutrition

This is currently a somewhat underdeveloped field but, as with lifestage feeding, the rabbit's increasing popularity is likely to lead to more research in this area and consequent recommendations concerning diet. Information available at the time of writing chiefly concentrates on the digestive and urinary tracts, together with the problem common to all domesticated species – obesity.

Obesity

Pet rabbits that are overweight are increasingly seen in veterinary surgeries. Lack of exercise is often a contributing factor, but overfeeding of concentrate rations is the main problem. Rabbits confined to small areas not only lack exercise but also tend to eat more because they are bored, so the problem is often related to both nutritional and environmental factors. Inappropriate sugary treats are also implicated.

In common with other animals, obesity in rabbits will place unnecessary stress on joints and decreases mobility. It can also contribute to the development of sore hocks (pododermatitis), when hair on the underside of the hocks is worn away and the skin becomes reddened and ulcerated. Secondary infections can then take hold and abscesses develop.

Rabbits can tolerate cold better than heat, preferring a temperature no higher than 15–16°C. Temperatures above this can lead to heat stress and in turn to respiratory problems. Obesity decreases the rabbit's ability to control body temperature during warm or hot weather and exacerbates the problem.

Overweight does often fail to breed, but those that do become pregnant are more susceptible to pregnancy toxaemia: the doe becomes inappetant and depressed and may abort. It is not unknown for convulsions and death to occur.

The major problem in obese rabbits is, however, interference with caecotrophy; quite simply the rabbit is too fat to be able to reach its anus and cannot therefore ingest the caecotrophs. These, because of their sticky nature, then cluster round the vent. This is doubtless uncomfortable but more seriously leaves the rabbit at risk of fly strike.

Restoring an obese rabbit to a more normal body weight is not easy – *prevention is better than cure*. In some cases less food, more exercise and a more interesting environment will be sufficient, in other cases a more drastic course of action will need to be taken. Starvation is not an option as the rabbit needs to continue to eat, but low-calorie, high-fibre foods should be offered. Concentrates should be phased out and replaced with more roughage in the form of green

> The major problem in obese rabbits is interference with caecotrophy.

vegetables and good-quality hay. Fresh water needs to be available at all times. The change in diet must be gradual because the sensitive digestive system must not be overwhelmed with new foods and mobilizing the rabbit's fat stores can lead to liver problems if too much is used at once.

Digestive system
Dental malocclusion

Malocclusion of the incisors is easily seen; that of the cheek teeth is less obvious, but none the less occurs frequently. The rabbit is usually inappetant, has lost weight, is drooling and often has a somewhat scruffy appearance due to the lack of grooming. If severely affected it may cease to eat caecotrophs and have a 'sticky bottom' as well as a dietary deficiency of protein and B complex vitamins.

Rabbit teeth are designed to cope with large quantities of coarse foods. The grinding action of the cheek teeth breaks down these foods to aid digestion but also erodes the surface of the teeth. Continual growth prevents the teeth from being completely worn away and the animal starving to death. When there is less work for the teeth, they continue to grow at the same rate but are worn down more slowly. Spikes may develop on the cheek teeth through uneven wear, which lacerate the gums and tongue; not surprisingly the rabbit is then reluctant to eat or groom. In severe cases the roots may be pushed backwards, giving a lumpy feel to the mandible and in the upper jaw impinging on the eye socket and displacing the nasolacrimal duct, so that many of these rabbits will have 'weepy eyes' as well as other symptoms. Abscesses are common.

Malocclusion is an inherited defect in some rabbits and affected animals should not be used for breeding. It is particularly common in dwarf rabbits, probably due to lack of jaw space. Other factors involved in malocclusion are lack of fibre and calcium deficiency. Feeding dry mixes reduces the amount of chewing; the food is more nutrient dense so less is eaten and components are often already crushed or cooked. Cereals contain more phosphorus than calcium, and when the diet contains a high proportion of cereal the calcium to phosphorus ratio is upset, leading to poor bone and dental quality and predisposing to malocclusion. Lack of sunlight reduces the amount of vitamin D available to the rabbit and affects the absorption of calcium.

Correction of malocclusion is difficult, so repeat the mantra – *prevention is better than cure*.

A well-balanced diet should include plenty of grass and other greenstuffs to encourage the correct side-to-side chewing action, and exposure to sunlight provided (best early morning and evening when the suns rays are not as strong). The addition of a good-quality vitamin and mineral supplement should be considered.

Enteropathies

Fibre is essential to maintain gastrointestinal tract (GIT) health. Insoluble (indigestible or non-fermentable) fibre encourages peristalsis throughout the gut and fermentable fibre helps maintain a healthy microbial population. Foods high in protein and/or simple carbohydrates are likely to upset the delicately balanced digestive system and lead to diarrhoea. Young rabbits are particularly susceptible to enteropathies. Raspberry, blackberry (bramble) or, in spring, young oak leaves are astringent and will help treat the resultant diarrhoea.

Mucoid enteropathy produces diarrhoea which contains mucus and has a jelly-like appearance. It occurs mainly in young rabbits but is seen in older animals. The affected rabbit is usually depressed and often bloated. Treatment is chiefly supportive but prognosis is guarded. Prevention includes the provision of adequate fibre and avoiding sudden dietary change.

Bloat

Bloat is caused by excess gas in the stomach and is usually associated with overfeeding of fresh foods, particularly those with a high water content. It is potentially fatal.

Probiotics

Probiotics are often recommended for rabbits with GIT upsets and several proprietary products are available. The best probiotic is said to be caecotrophs from another rabbit – fine in theory, but in practice not easy! First, caecotrophs are rarely found lying about, so good timing and the cooperation of a friendly rabbit are essential. Secondly, persuading a depressed rabbit to eat something that is handled with distaste by the owner, is probably cold and presumably smells of another rabbit, needs craft and cunning.

Urinary system

Rabbits suffer from urolithiasis and cystitis, which may be dietary related. Symptoms are similar to those in other species. Rabbits excrete higher levels of calcium through the kidneys than other mammals, so calcium carbonate crystals in the bladder can be regarded as normal. When these form into stones they may lodge in the neck of the bladder or in the urethra, causing problems and requiring surgical removal. Excess calcium in the diet will exacerbate the problem, so should be avoided. Alfalfa, dandelions and spinach are all high in calcium.

The endocrine system

Diabetes mellitus is not common but can occur in some older rabbits and is said to be more common in New Zealand White rabbits. Injecting insulin is impractical, so treatment is dependent on diet. Simple sugars in fruits and young, growing greenstuffs should be avoided and adequate levels of fibre provided.

Summing up

The origins of the hutch and cereal feeding were to produce a rabbit which fattened quickly and was ready for the pot as soon as possible – not exactly the intention of the current pet rabbit owner. The provision of a diet as close as possible to that of a wild rabbit, with a small amount of good-quality concentrate to compensate for inadequate browsing areas, will enable the pet rabbit to lead a long and enjoyable life and provide the owner with companionship over a number of years.

RODENTS

The remainder of the small furries currently kept as pets belong to the order of mammals known as Rodentia. Rodents are gnawing animals that often hoard food. Chinchillas and guinea-pigs are strict herbivores, while the other small furries will consume varying amounts of animal protein. Many of these rodents are fed a diet low in protein and sometimes fail to reach their genetic potential for growth because of this protein shortage.

Although most small rodents are very active and, with a high surface area to bodyweight ratio, have high energy requirements, when kept as pets they spend less time and energy foraging for food than they are obliged to do in the wild and obesity is thus always a threat. This should be guarded against for all the usual reasons.

These small rodents, with the exception of some hamsters, are sociable animals and are happier living with at least one other member of the same species. The presence of a companion encourages them to be more active and helps prevent excessive eating by keeping boredom at bay.

Proprietary rations are available for these pets but home-made diets are also easily prepared for most species. Rodents should be weaned onto a diet containing as wide a variety of foods as possible, as the adult's diet tends to reflect what it received as a youngster.

Some foods are best avoided or fed only in small quantities to any rodent. Chief examples of these are sunflower seeds and peanuts. Sunflower seeds are well liked by all rodents and will be eaten in preference to many other foods; unfortunately they are high in fat and low in calcium so form a far from ideal diet. Peanuts are also enjoyed but are high in fat and when taken into food stores will often develop mould growth, which may be toxic and will contaminate other foods in the store.

Peanut shells when chewed can break into spiky pieces which will scratch the mouth and pouches of rodents, so are best avoided.

CHINCHILLAS

Chinchillas originate from South America where they live in the mountains and high valleys of Argentina, Bolivia and Chile. They are active during early evening and through the night, usually avoiding the higher day temperatures in burrows or rock crevices. Chinchillas are more difficult to keep as pets than other small furries as they have more specific requirements. The preferred temperature for chinchillas is between 10 and 15°C, although they can tolerate temperatures up to 25°C. Above this they are susceptible to heat stroke. Sudden changes in temperature should be avoided. Dry cold, as in their natural environment, is tolerated better than the warmer but damper conditions of a British winter.

They need well-ventilated, draught-free quarters which are not in direct sunlight and with provision to hide away during the day if they wish to do so.

Chinchillas are more sensitive to humidity than most rodents. Too low and they are susceptible to respiratory disease, too high and they become stressed; around 70% humidity seems to be best for them.

In their natural habitat, vegetation is sparse and often of fairly poor quality. They eat grass, fruit, leaves and bark, most of which are high in fibre. Their digestive system is therefore designed to cope with a high-fibre, low-energy content diet. They have a large stomach and an enlarged caecum to accommodate the large quantities of fibre ingested. Caecal pellets are produced and eaten, providing a source of B vitamins and protein. Adult chinchillas require protein levels of around 15%, while fibre should be twice this at 30%. Young animals, pregnant and lactating females and animals recovering from illness, require extra protein.

Some chinchillas appear to have very specific nutritional needs, including a dietary source of pre-formed vitamin A and arachidonic acid, which may indicate that they are not quite the strict herbivores we believe them to be. These special needs are, however, best supplied within a proprietary diet. These are available either in pelleted form or as a mix of various ingredients. When chinchilla diets are not available, a diet designed for guinea-pigs may be fed, although this is not ideal.

Vegetables and fruit may be added, but in very small quantities and only once or twice weekly. One-eighth of a medium-sized apple is suggested or similarly small quantities of carrot or celery. Chinchillas love raisins but should be given no more than two daily. They help prevent constipation and are useful for medication should it be necessary. Fat levels should be low and, for this reason, nuts and sunflower seeds should not be fed. Good-quality hay and fresh water should always be available.

> Chinchillas love raisins but should be given no more than two daily.

The daily ration should be split into two equal portions and fed morning and evening. Pregnant and lactating females will benefit from ad lib feeding, particularly during late pregnancy when stomach capacity is reduced by the enlarged uterus. Chinchilla kits are born fully developed, placing extra nutritional demands on the mother, so an adequate diet is essential.

Clinical nutrition

Conditions influenced by diet include:

- malocclusion
- diarrhoea
- constipation
- bloat.

Malocclusion

Like rabbits, the teeth of chinchillas are open rooted to cope with the wear placed on them by fibrous foods and, again like rabbits, problems can arise when the pet chinchilla has insufficient fibre in its diet.

The dental formula is I1/1, C0/0, P1/1, M3/3.

Chinchillas with maloccluded teeth will be inappetent and often drooling – 'slobbers'. The molar teeth may develop spikes which should be trimmed when necessary, but there may be root overgrowth through the mandible and maxilla. Increasing the fibre content of the diet will increase the wear on the teeth and help prevent spikes reforming. Branches and twigs of hawthorn or fruit trees should be provided to give additional chewing exercise. Pumice stone will be gnawed, helping to keep the incisors trimmed.

When malocclusion is severe, puréed foods may need to be fed but these will not cure the problem and removal of the affected teeth should be considered.

Dietary imbalances in the calcium to phosphorus ratio can lead to abnormalities in the formation of the teeth. This is particularly a problem in lactating females when their requirement for calcium increases and supplementation may be necessary at this time.

Diarrhoea

Normal chinchilla droppings are elongated, firm and slightly moist.

Diarrhoea, when the faecal pellets are watery and sometimes contain blood and mucus, has several causes, including overfeeding and sudden changes in the diet. Hay and water only should be fed until the droppings return to normal.

Constipation

Constipation produces small faecal pellets, which are hard and dry. The water supply should be checked as constipation can be due to lack of fluids. Adding fresh foods to the diet, e.g. apple, carrot, dandelion or groundsel, will often help, as do the two raisins a day. The chinchilla should also be encouraged to exercise more.

Bloat

Bloat is often associated with a change in diet, particularly when fibre levels fall or when fruits and greenstuffs are fed in larger than normal quantities. Gastric stasis allows fermentation to take place and gas accumulates, distending the stomach and causing dyspnoea. It is potentially fatal.

Dietary changes should be made slowly and fibre levels kept around 30%.

Probiotics

Probiotics may be helpful in re-establishing normal gut flora after digestive upsets. Live yoghurt or proprietary products may be used, or caecotrophs from another healthy chinchilla, but this carries the same reservations as for rabbits.

CHIPMUNKS

Chipmunks are relative newcomers to the pet scene and although hand-reared chipmunks or young ones acquired before 3 months of age can, with patience, become very tame, adults are very suspicious of humans, are difficult to handle and have a very sharp bite. They are best regarded at present as captive animals rather than domesticated pets.

Chipmunks are related to squirrels, are very active and need space to run, burrow and climb. Most of the chipmunks kept as pets are Siberian chipmunks and in the wild live in burrows. They are active during the day and hibernate in winter. Chipmunks kept outdoors in Britain may also hibernate and will require extra stores of food to prepare for this. Some may stay in their sleeping quarters on cold days but emerge to forage on warmer days. At these times they will appreciate small quantities of fresh foods, but only dry foods should be offered for storage to prevent deterioration and mould growth.

Chipmunks are omnivorous, hoard food and practise coprophagy. In the wild they eat fruit, nuts, berries, grains, green vegetation, weeds and bark. They will also eat grubs, insects, birds' eggs and chicks when available. Carrion will sometimes be eaten.

They normally forage over wide areas and in captivity may find food too easily, leading to lack of exercise, boredom, overeating and obesity. Dry food can be scattered or hidden in the cage litter. Branches from fruit trees, hawthorn, beech or birch should be provided for climbing and gnawing and food can be lodged in crevices in these to encourage foraging.

Chipmunks in captivity should be fed as wide a variety of foods as possible. An adult will consume around 30 g dry weight daily and this should be given in two equal portions. Food not eaten immediately will be stored, often in the nest box. Owners should be aware of the site of the food store and check it regularly as fresh food placed in there may become mouldy and contaminate other foodstuff. Undue interference with the store may discourage the animal from using it and it will then permanently store food in its cheek pouches. When this happens the pouch linings are often damaged and may become infected. Fresh foods are best fed with care and in small quantities, which usually ensures they are eaten immediately rather than stored.

> Chipmunks in captivity should be fed as wide as variety of foods as possible.

It is often difficult to find proprietary rations specifically prepared for chipmunks, but hamster mixes can be used. These should be supplemented with foods of animal origin such as hard-boiled egg or small amounts of tinned dog food. Wild herbs and weeds can be fed after washing and drying. Sunflower seeds are liked but should be offered sparingly because of their high fat content.

Young animals, and pregnant and lactating females, require extra protein, which can be offered in the form of extra hard-boiled egg, cheese, milk powder, crickets or mealworms. Mealworms are low in calcium and high in phosphorus, so dusting them with bonemeal prior to feeding will improve the ratio. Foods prepared for insectivorous birds can also be fed.

Wheat germ should be sprinkled on dry foods and offered to breeding stock to increase dietary levels of vitamin E, as low levels may lead to infertility.

Clinical nutrition

Conditions influenced by diet include:

- malocclusion
- dental caries
- diarrhoea.

Malocclusion

The dental formula is I1/1, C0/0, P0/0, M3/3.

The incisors grow continually, so chipmunks need plenty of gnawing exercise to keep the teeth trimmed. Dog biscuits and nuts in their hard shells, together with branches and twigs, provide this exercise. They will chew any wood in the cage, including the framework, and a close watch should be kept on this for possible escape holes being formed. As many chipmunks are housed outdoors, escapees are much less easily recaptured.

Dental caries

Dental caries, which destroys the tooth enamel, occurs in chipmunks when their diet contains too many foods high in simple carbohydrates or acids. Dental caries causes pain and salivation and the condition can be prevented if the offending foods are avoided.

Dental caries occur in chipmunks when their diet contains too many foods high in simple carbohydrates or acids.

Diarrhoea

Diarrhoea in chipmunks is usually due either to sudden changes in the diet or eating fresh food which has 'gone off'. Astringent raspberry and blackberry leaves are beneficial, but other fresh foods should not be fed until the problem resolves. Dry mix, hay and water only should be offered.

GERBILS

The gerbil species commonly kept as a pet in Britain is the Mongolian gerbil, which is native to desert and semi-desert areas of Mongolia and northern China, where the summers are hot and winters cold and dry. The preferred temperature for these gerbils is between 15 and 25°C, with a relative low humidity. In the wild they will burrow underground to avoid extremes of temperatures or high humidity (heat tolerance decreases as humidity increases); this burrowing habit should be allowed for when they are kept as pets. Their natural habitats are areas of sparse vegetation and very low rainfall. As a result, gerbils are able to conserve fluid, producing a very concentrated urine and faeces which are normally very dry. Despite this, fresh clean water should always be available

Gerbils are omnivores rather than strict herbivores and in their natural habitat they eat seeds, grain, green vegetation and roots. They will also eat small quantities of insects and grubs. They do not usually practise coprophagy.

They live in groups and are active during the day. When kept as pets they need plenty of room to exercise and furnishings such as cardboard tubes to provide interest and prevent boredom. Hiding food in the cage litter encourages foraging activity.

They require protein levels of around 16% and fat levels of around 5%. Breeding animals require a higher than maintenance level of protein and fat. Animal protein is particularly important at this stage and can be provided in the form of hard-boiled egg, milk powder, cottage cheese, yoghurt or mealworms (dusted in bonemeal before feeding).

> Gerbils require protein levels around 16% and fat levels of around 5%.

The digestive system of the gerbil is less well designed to cope with large amounts of fibre, so this needs to be lower than in diets for rabbits, chinchillas and guinea-pigs. Hay should be provided, although this is often used for nest material rather than being eaten. Coarse hay will damage the gerbil's cheek pouches, so good-quality soft hay should be chosen.

Small quantities of fresh food can be offered each day but should be removed if not eaten to prevent mould growth in food stores. Wholegrain bread or crackers can be fed.

Clinical nutrition

Conditions influenced by diet include:

- malocclusion
- diarrhoea

- constipation
- diabetes mellitus
- kidney disease.

Malocclusion

Gerbils have continually growing incisors and need hard foods to prevent overgrowth. Dog biscuits can be provided, along with the usual branches and twigs.

Diarrhoea

Diarrhoea may be caused by sudden changes of food or eating stale foods. Dry foods and water only should be fed until the condition resolves. When the diarrhoea is severe, electrolyte solutions should be made available as well as water and this can be syringe fed. Raspberry or blackberry leaves, dry arrowroot biscuits and wholemeal toast will help clear the diarrhoea. Probiotics should be given to help restore the normal gut flora.

Constipation

When the animal is constipated there are fewer than normal faecal pellets produced and, in some cases, none at all. The abdomen may be swollen and the affected animal will appear uncomfortable. Green foods, particularly dandelion leaves, are useful, although they should be used with care when they are not normally fed.

Diabetes mellitus

Polyuria and polydipsia are often seen in older gerbils. In obese animals this may be due to diabetes mellitus. Fruits and young tender leaves should not be fed.

> Polyuria and polydipsia are often seen in older gerbils.

Kidney disease

When the gerbil is not obese and has a history of recent weight loss, the likely cause of polyuria and polydipsia is chronic kidney disease. There is little that can be done from a dietary point of view, but electrolyte solutions should be offered in addition to water and supplements of the water-soluble vitamins should be given.

GUINEA-PIGS

Guinea-pigs (or cavies) originate from South America, where they live on grassland and the lower slopes of mountains in Argentina, Brazil, Peru and Uruguay, and were kept as food animals and pets by the Incas. They were brought to Europe by early explorers and became popular as pets and show animals from the eighteenth century onwards.

In their natural habitat they eat grass, other green-stuffs, fruits and seeds. They are strict herbivores and practise coprophagy. They are active during the day, although they are often most active at dusk.

Guinea-pigs require relatively high levels of protein (around 18%) and around 15% of fibre in their diet. Fat levels should be less than 5%. Unlike most mammals but in common with humans, guinea-pigs cannot synthesize vitamin C, so require a supply in their diet. They are also only able to store this vitamin for short periods, so require 10 mg per kg daily. Pregnant sows require twice this amount. Fresh, recently growing foods will contain sufficient levels of vitamin C, but those that have been picked several days previously, e.g. shop-bought cabbage, will have low levels. Broccoli has higher than average levels. Vitamin C can be provided in the drinking water. Ascorbic acid breaks down quickly in water, so a fresh solution should be mixed each day. Breakdown is accelerated in the presence of organic material or metals other than stainless steel (many drinking bottles have non-stainless steel nozzles). Administering an ascorbic acid tablet direct is a better method.

> Guinea-pigs require relatively high levels of protein (around 18%) and around 15% of fibre in their diet.

Good-quality guinea-pig foods are supplemented with vitamin C but should be stored in cool dry conditions and used quickly. When stored for long periods the vitamin levels will fall.

Grass can form a major part of the guinea-pig's diet and other fresh foods can be offered in small quantities daily. Guinea-pigs that have wintered indoors eating chiefly dry foods, should initially have limited access to grass in the spring. Periods of access can be gradually lengthened. Hay or good-quality oat straw and fresh water should always be available.

Young stock and breeding stock will require extra protein, and feeding a good-quality guinea-pig mix ad lib should allow for this. Other adults are best fed their daily ration in two equal portions.

Guinea-pigs give birth to offspring that are fully developed, their eyes are open and they are covered with hair. They are able to walk soon after birth. The sow's requirements for protein, energy and calcium are high in pregnancy and the provision of a good, well-balanced diet throughout this time is essential to avoid the dangers of pregnancy toxaemia. The addition of small amounts of glucose to the drinking water and calcium supplementation during the last 7–10 days of pregnancy and first week of lactation will also help prevent this problem and eclampsia which sometimes occurs in older sows.

Bran mashes are sometimes recommended for pregnant sows but should be used with care because of the low calcium, high phosphorus content.

Clinical nutrition

Conditions influenced by diet include:

- vitamin and mineral deficiencies
- malocclusion
- gastric dilation
- diarrhoea
- caecal impaction
- renal failure
- urolithiasis
- diabetes mellitus.

Vitamin and mineral deficiencies

Guinea-pigs are susceptible to disorders caused by imbalances in the calcium to phosphorus ratio of their diet; levels of vitamin D, magnesium and potassium are also important to ensure adequate mineralization of bones and teeth. In older animals these imbalances may lead to deposition of calcium in soft tissue, including the kidneys, heart and gastric wall. This interferes with normal function of the organs and is ultimately fatal. A good well-balanced diet should be fed throughout life.

Skin conditions are often due to, or are worsened by, hypovitaminosis C and correction of levels of this vitamin in the diet will usually see an improvement.

Malocclusion

The dental formula is I1/1, C0/0, P1/1, M3/3.

As with the rabbit and chinchilla, all the teeth grow continually. Guinea-pigs require roughage in the diet to keep the teeth worn evenly. Overgrowth of the incisors is usually obvious but cheek teeth should be checked if the animal is inappetent and drooling. Sharp spikes may develop on the molars which can lacerate the gums and tongue. In severe cases the tongue may be trapped and the guinea-pig is unable to swallow. Dental problems are more frequent in older animals.

Prevention, as usual, involves the provision of hard foods, hay and branches or twigs to chew on.

Some malocclusions of the incisors are due to an undershot jaw and these animals will need extra attention paid to their teeth. Malocclusion in guinea-pigs is often hereditary and affected animals should not be used for breeding.

Gastric dilation

Sudden changes in the diet and overfeeding of green foods will cause digestive problems leading to diarrhoea and/or gaseous distension of the bowel. Gastric dilation is often accompanied by volvulus and will require surgical intervention if it is not to prove fatal.

Dietary changes must be made slowly and feeding fresh foods that are wet or frosted should be avoided.

Diarrhoea

Diarrhoea in guinea-pigs often has dietary causes as outlined above. Moulds, which may grow on both fresh and dry foods but especially on hay, cause diarrhoea, so all food should be carefully checked before feeding. Guinea-pigs with diarrhoea should be fed only on dry food, good-quality hay and water until the condition resolves.

Caecal impaction

Caecal impaction can occur in guinea-pigs, particularly older ones who have loss of muscle tone. Surgical intervention may be necessary. Adequate levels of fibre should be provided and overfeeding avoided to lessen the risk of this problem developing.

Renal failure

Beetroot (leaves), spinach and dock leaves contain oxalic acid, the percentage increasing as the stems age and turn woody. If large amounts of these are eaten, oxalic acid poisoning can result, leading to acute renal failure and death.

Urolithiasis

Some degree of crystalluria is normal but calculi may form on occasion and cause problems, particularly in males. Predisposing factors are nutritional imbalances, bacterial infections and low fluid intake.

Surgical removal of bladder stones is recommended but small calculi may dissolve if the urine is acidified. Apple and beetroot both have a high acid content and may reduce the pH of the urine sufficiently.

Diabetes mellitus

Diabetes mellitus occurs occasionally in guinea-pigs. Treatment with insulin is impractical, so dietary control should be attempted. Fruits and other foods likely to contain high levels of simple carbohydrates should be avoided and increasing fibre levels will help even out blood glucose levels.

Polyuria associated with diabetes mellitus leads to increased loss of water-soluble vitamins and extra ascorbic acid, and supplements of the B complex vitamins may be required. Polyuria may also cause urine scald; absorbent bedding which is changed regularly will help prevent this.

HAMSTERS

The Syrian (or Golden) hamster is one of the most popular pets in Britain, but species of dwarf hamsters are also kept, principally the Russian and Chinese hamsters.

Syrian hamsters originate from the desert areas of Syria where they live in deep burrows which protect them from the heat of the day. They are solitary animals in the wild and when kept as pets should be kept singly. Adult Syrian hamsters can vary in size from 85 to 140 g, with the female usually larger than the male. In contrast, the dwarf hamsters weigh around 40 g as adults. A fourth species, the Roborovski hamster, is even smaller with adults weighing about 35 g.

Russian hamsters originate from central Asia, Russia and Siberia. In their natural habitat they live in small groups, one male with several females, and like company when kept as pets. They can be kept in pairs or in groups, as in the wild.

Roborovski hamsters come from Mongolia; they also are social animals and are best kept in pairs.

Chinese hamsters, originate from northern China. They are less sociable than Russian hamsters but will live in pairs if introduced when young. Chinese hamsters belong to the long-tailed group of hamster, unlike the Russian and Roborovski hamsters which have short tails.

Although these species of hamster originate in different parts of the world, they all have similar habitats – deserts or other barren areas. They are omnivorous, eating seeds, grain, green vegetation and fruits when available, together with insects and grubs. They are chiefly crepuscular or nocturnal animals, are coprophagic and hoard food.

Hamsters kept as pets are often short of animal protein; hamster mix should be supplemented with hard-boiled egg, cheese, dried milk powder, small amounts of dog or cat food, mealworms or foods designed for insectivorous birds. As always, young animals, and pregnant and lactating females, have a higher requirement for protein (around 24%). Other adults will need around 18% protein. Dwarf hamsters must be fed with care as they require very small amounts of food and it is easy to overfeed them, leading to obesity and all its attendant problems.

All species of hamster are hoarders of food and these stores should be inspected regularly for signs of mould. Fresh food should only be fed in small amounts; this way it is eaten rather than stored. Foods

> Hamsters are chiefly crepuscular or nocturnal animals, are coprophagic and hoard food.

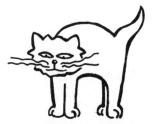

> **NB!**
> Dwarf hamsters are easy to overfeed.

with a high moisture content such as lettuce and cucumber are best avoided. Broccoli, pear, apple, parsley and carrot are more suitable. Small quantities of washed and dried wild plants (as for rabbits) can be fed to adults, but should be fed with care to young stock.

Sharp foods, e.g. seed husks, may damage the lining of the cheek pouches and are best avoided.

Clinical nutrition

Conditions influenced by diet include:

- cage paralysis
- malocclusion
- dental caries
- diarrhoea
- constipation
- chronic renal failure
- urolithiasis
- diabetes mellitus.

Cage paralysis

Hamsters confined to too small an area and with low levels of vitamins D and E in their diet are prone to this condition, appearing stiff, reluctant to move and often dragging their hind legs. Feeding a proprietary balanced mix should provide adequate vitamin levels and the affected animal should be moved to a bigger cage or provided with more opportunity to exercise outside its existing cage.

Malocclusion

The dental formula is I1/1, C0/0, P0/0, M3/3.

The incisors are open rooted and continue to grow throughout life, so hamsters should have plenty of material to gnaw on. Hard foods, including dog biscuits and dry wholemeal macaroni, can be offered, along with wood from non-poisonous trees.

Dental caries

Dental caries is common in hamsters fed foods high in simple carbohydrates. They will quickly develop a preference for these foods, so they should be avoided or severely restricted.

Diarrhoea

Diarrhoea is often associated with sudden dietary changes or eating stale or mouldy food. Only dry food (arrowroot biscuits are helpful) and water should be offered until the diarrhoea is resolved. It is important to remove the stored food, as this may be the source of the contamination.

Constipation

Constipation can occur when hamsters have no access to water while they are offered a dry diet. Weanlings are particularly prone to this condition and care should be taken to ensure that they can reach water bottles.

Small quantities of dandelion, groundsel or lettuce can be fed to relieve the condition, or one drop of liquid paraffin three times a day administered to the affected animal.

Chronic renal failure

Older hamsters may develop chronic renal failure (too high protein levels fed to adults may predispose to kidney problems or they may develop as a consequence of heat stroke) and show the usual clinical signs of polyuria and polydipsia. Adding boiled rice to the diet and reducing protein levels may be helpful.

Diabetes mellitus

Diabetes mellitus occurs in Chinese hamsters as an inherited condition and is usually evident by the age of 3 months. These animals should not be used for breeding. Diabetes mellitus is seen less frequently in other species of hamster.

Dietary restrictions will help manage blood glucose levels and prolong the hamster's life. Sweet foods, fruits and young leaves should not be fed and a slight increase in fibre levels is usually beneficial. Most affected hamsters will lose weight.

The polyuria associated with diabetes mellitus will require the use of absorbent bedding which will need to be changed at least daily.

MICE AND RATS

Mice and rats have similar nutritional requirements and so may be considered together. Both of these species probably originate from the Far East but have been present in Britain since at least the seventeenth century. In the wild they eat seeds and grain, but they are opportunist omnivores and will eat almost anything which is the remotest bit edible, even though this is not necessarily good for them. Chocolate designed for human consumption is toxic to rats when eaten in quantity.

They are primarily nocturnal but, when kept as pets, can be active for short periods during the day, resting or sleeping between these bursts of activity.

Mice are social animals and should not be kept singly. To avoid endless offspring, two or three females should be kept together. Rats may be kept singly but then require a lots of attention from their owner. They may be kept in same sex pairs if introduced when young.

Proprietary mixes are available for both rats and mice and these provide a balanced complete diet. Small amounts of fresh food and animal protein can be added to provide extra variety. Home-made diets can be based on oats (whole or crushed) and wholemeal bread, toasted or dried to encourage gnawing. Small amounts of fresh foods provide extra vitamins and minerals. Animal protein should also be offered and good-quality hay provided. This will chiefly be used for bedding but some will be eaten. Fresh water should always be available.

Protein levels for young animals and breeding stock should be fairly high at around 24%, while other adult mice and rats require only 15%; protein levels above these can lead to skin problems.

Obesity is a common problem in pet mice and rats due to inadequate exercise.

Clinical nutrition

Given a balanced diet, mice and rats are usually healthy animals but some conditions occur which are influenced by diet including:

- malocclusion
- dental caries
- diarrhoea
- chronic renal failure.

Malocclusion

In common with other rodents, mice and rats have continually growing incisors and require adequate supplies of hard materials to gnaw on.

Dental caries

Dental caries occurs in rats that develop a liking for sweet treats. Cakes and sweet biscuits should not be fed, except occasionally as a treat.

Diarrhoea

Diarrhoea can occur with overfeeding, too sudden changes of diet or eating contaminated foods. It is much more common in young animals. Diarrhoea in older mice and rats is unlikely to be associated with diet. Treatment is, as usual, dry food (including arrowroot biscuits) and water only.

Chronic renal failure

Chronic renal failure (CRF) is common in older rats fed on high-protein diets. For this reason, protein levels in non-breeding stock should be reduced once the animals reach 3 months of age. Rats with CRF may benefit from a reduced protein diet and added boiled rice.

FERRETS

And so back to carnivores. Ferrets have a long association with humans as working animals, but more recently are establishing a reputation as intelligent pets. They are very adaptable and can live either indoors or outdoors, but require secure accommodation to prevent escapes and limit their chewing to safe objects. They are burrowing animals and ideally provision should be made for this habit wherever they are housed.

Ferrets are sociable animals and are best kept in pairs or small groups. They should have a draught-free shelter to protect them from unfavourable temperatures, with adequate ventilation throughout their quarters.

Ferrets have been kept in captivity for centuries and are not found living in the wild except for a few escapees, so assumptions have to be made about their natural diet. They are related to and probably descended from the European polecat and also related to mink, stoats and weasels. These small carnivores are all efficient hunters and in their natural habitats eat voles, mice, shrews, squirrels, birds and rabbits. They will also take eggs and insects as well as some fruits and berries. It is safe to assume that feral ferrets eat the same diet. In captivity their curiosity may lead them to eat unsuitable foods and those kept as pets may be offered biscuits and sweets which will be eaten, but are inappropriate. Theobromine found in chocolate for human consumption is toxic to ferrets, as it also is for dogs and rats.

The ferret's wild relatives are mainly nocturnal; ferrets spend a lot of their time sleeping but are usually active around meal times, regardless of when these are.

Under natural conditions, prey is eaten whole, ensuring that all the required vitamins and minerals are consumed. They are obligate carnivores and require animal protein in their diet, but ferrets kept as pets may be fed muscle meat alone; this forms an incomplete diet. Young ferrets reared on all-meat diets without calcium supplementation can develop osteodystrophy. The calcium to phosphorus ratio should be 1:1. Their natural diet includes little fibre and their digestive system is not designed to cope with more than 5% fibre.

Specialist ferret foods are now available but ferrets can also be fed dry cat food, either straight from the packet or slightly moistened. They have high protein requirements and dog food usually has inadequate protein levels.

Ferrets have a short gut transit time, so the food must be highly digestible. They should be fed at least twice daily; young and older ferrets should be fed smaller meals more often.

Water should be provided in heavy dishes which cannot be easily overturned; even so they will play with the water and the dishes should be checked, cleaned and refilled frequently.

Food and water should not be given in galvanized containers as these 'leak' zinc into the food or water. Levels of zinc around 500 ppm are toxic to ferrets.

Male ferrets are larger than females and this difference is apparent early, from about 6 weeks of age. This may lead to worries among novice ferret breeders that some kits are doing less well than others.

Lifestage feeding

Young growing ferrets and pregnant and lactating females have a minimum requirement of 35% protein and 20% fat (30% for lactating jills) in their diet.

Ferret kits are voracious feeders and the jill needs to produce large quantities of milk, particularly so with a large litter. To be able to do this she needs plenty of energy-dense food and water. Jills may also require a balanced vitamin and mineral supplement to guard against hypocalcaemia, which is occasionally seen at the time of peak demand for milk, 3 weeks after parturition. Non-breeding adults require a diet lower in protein (30%) and fat (18%).

Clinical nutrition

Conditions influenced by diet include:

- dental problems
- gastroenteritis
- chronic interstitial nephritis
- urolithiasis.

Dental problems

Ferret kits are born toothless. Deciduous teeth erupt between 2 and 4 weeks and are shed by 10 weeks. The permanent teeth start to erupt at 6 weeks and are

normally all present by the age of 10 weeks.
The dental formulae are:

Deciduous – I4/3, C1/1, P3/3.
Permanent – I3/3, C1/1, P3/3, M1/2.

Dental calculus will develop when ferrets are fed on moist food alone; they require tough meat, dry food or hard biscuit to maintain the teeth in good condition.

Gastroenteritis

Gastritis and gastroenteritis occur in ferrets for a variety of reasons. If the animal is vomiting, food should be withheld for 6–12 hours and then a bland food offered little and often. It should be easily digested, high in carbohydrate and low in fibre – the traditional chicken and boiled rice can be tried. Bland diets should also be fed when the ferret is suffering from diarrhoea.

Normal food can be gradually reintroduced when the symptoms resolve.

Chronic interstitial nephritis

Renal disease, except for chronic interstitial nephritis, is uncommon in ferrets, despite their high-protein diet. It has been suggested that older ferrets (more than 3 or 4 years) should be fed a diet containing less protein to reduce the effects of this condition.

Urolithiasis

Ferrets fed diets high in plant proteins are predisposed to developing cystic calculi, although other factors, e.g. urinary tract infections, are also involved. Struvite are the commonest crystals found; animal proteins usually produce an acidic urine which dissolves struvite crystals, while plant proteins produce a more alkaline urine which precipitates out these crystals. Diet therefore plays a large part in the control of urolithiasis.

HAND REARING SMALL FURRIES

At times it may be necessary to hand rear the young of this group of pets. Some species are easier to rear than others. All will benefit from even a short time spent suckling their mother, as the colostrum provides passive immunity to the neonate and greatly increases the chances of its survival. The milk substitute should be fed at body temperature and hygiene is all important.

A small syringe may be used or kitten feeding bottles. When teats are used, the neonate tends to drink more and therefore may need feeding less often. The neonate should be held upright to enable it to swallow easily; milk should not be forced into the mouth as this may cause inhalation pneumonia which is usually fatal; teat feeding is safer than using a syringe.

The amount to be fed is often found by trial and error; it is best to start with very small amounts and gradually increase them. After feeding, the neonate should be stimulated to urinate and defecate, although by the time they are 1 week old this is often unnecessary.

It is important to establish and stick to a routine and the neonates should be weighed regularly to check on their progress.

Rabbits

Rabbit kits are born blind and hairless. Orphaned kits can be fostered by other does and are accepted best during the first few days after birth. The doe normally only feeds her young once or at most twice a day and she may not come into milk until 24 hours after the birth, so owners should not interfere too early.

Hand rearing is possible but difficult. Feline milk substitute can be used, to which a multivitamin supplement and a probiotic should be added. The does milk is higher in fat than the feline milk substitute, so it is necessary to feed the kits more often than the doe does – three to four times a day is sufficient.

Hay can be offered from 3 weeks, followed by solid food as the kits grow. They should be fully weaned by 6–7 weeks old.

Chinchillas

Chinchilla young are born with their eyes open and fully furred. Orphaned or rejected kits may be fostered onto another chinchilla or they can be hand reared. Canine milk substitutes may be used or evaporated milk diluted with equal parts of cooled boiled water, and they should be fed initially about every 2 hours. This dilution may be too rich for some kits and in these cases the evaporated milk can be diluted further: two parts water to one part evaporated milk, with a small amount of glucose powder added.

Small amounts of baby cereal, vitamin drops and a probiotic can be added after the first week and the intervals between feeds gradually increased. The kits will start to take solid food at 7–10 days but will not be fully weaned until they are 7 or 8 weeks old.

Chipmunks

Chipmunks are born blind and hairless and remain in the nest box for about 5 weeks. Hand rearing young chipmunks is possible after the age of 1 week; prior to this it is impractical. Initially, evaporated milk diluted one part milk with two parts cooled boiled water should be given every 4 hours. From 2 weeks of age, small amounts of baby cereal and a probiotic can be added to the dilution. The intervals between feeds can be gradually increased; at 3 weeks old they will only need three feeds daily.

Gerbils

Gerbils are born blind and hairless. They start to eat solid food at around 2 weeks old and are fully weaned a week to 10 days later. Weanlings must be able to reach water bottles.

Orphaned young may be fostered by another female but hand rearing is impractical.

Guinea-pigs

Guinea-piglets are born fully developed, miniatures of their parents. They will start eating hay from day 2 and piglets orphaned after 3 days will survive without help. Those orphaned at or soon after birth may be fostered onto another sow or hand reared. They are born with sufficient energy reserves to last 12 hours, which allows time to find a foster mother or make other arrangements. Canine milk replacer can be used and fed every 2 hours initially. They should be encouraged to take solid food as soon as possible and milk can be decreased as consumption of solids increases. They are fully weaned at 3 weeks of age.

Hamsters

Hamsters are born blind, hairless and with undeveloped limbs. They will start to eat solids at about 10 days old and are fully weaned between 3 and 4 weeks of age. Fostering orphan hamsters is rarely successful and hand rearing impractical.

Mice and rats

Mice and rat pups are born blind and hairless. They are fully weaned by 3–4 weeks old. Hand rearing is impractical.

Ferrets

Ferret kits are born with their eyes and ears closed but are covered with a fine hair coat and stay in the nest for the first 2–3 weeks. They start to eat solid food as they emerge from the nest and are fully weaned at 6–8 weeks old. Orphaned kits may be hand reared once they are 7–10 days old; prior to this they are best fostered onto another jill. Canine or feline milk replacer may be used, but as this is lower in fat than ferret milk, one part single cream should be added to three parts milk replacer. It should be fed initially every 2 hours but decreasing to three or four times daily at 3 weeks old. The kits should be offered solid food from 3 weeks and can be weaned from 5 weeks onwards, provided that they are eating solid food adequately.

PRE- AND POST-OP FEEDING

The appearance of small furries on the op list no longer raises eyebrows, nor quick glances at the calendar (no, it's not April 1st). The advent of new anaesthetics has lowered the risk involved and as survival rates increase, owners are more willing to have these pets operated on.

Sharing the op list with dogs and cats does not mean however that pre-anaesthetic protocols should be the same. Dogs and cats are generally starved for 12 hours prior to an op. For small furries, with their high metabolic rates and low reserves of protein and energy, 12 hours without food is a dangerously long time. Their bodies will have entered a catabolic state, increasing the anaesthetic risk and prolonging recovery time. In addition, starvation is unnecessary because rabbits and the small rodents are unable to vomit or regurgitate, thus removing the risk of aspiration of stomach contents into the lungs.

When rabbits, chinchillas and guinea-pigs have eaten a large meal, the full stomach may impinge on the thoracic cavity, particularly when the animal is in dorsal recumbency, reducing lung capacity. Withholding food for 2–3 hours prior to the operation will ensure that the stomach is not overfull and raising the chest above the abdomen during surgery will take pressure off the thorax.

The other small rodents should not be starved. In all cases water should be available up to the time of surgery, as dehydration is a significant risk factor.

Ferrets are able to vomit but, because they have a rapid gut transit time, it is not necessary to starve them for more than 6 hours. Ferrets over 3 years old should be starved for no more than 4 hours. The owner would normally feed a small meal on the morning of the operation.

It is important to bear in mind the time of the animal's last meal when deciding on the order of the ops (remember to ask the owner when this was when admitting the animal). If the fasting period is to be overlong, the patient should be encouraged to eat a small meal while waiting.

Familiar food will be more readily accepted than the unfamiliar (and possibly stale) food kept on the top shelf of the kennel room. The owner should be asked to bring a small amount of their pet's normal food with them and also asked if it has any favourite 'treats', as these can be a helpful stimulant to the appetite post-op (even if shortbread biscuits should not normally be fed!).

In some practices, operating on these small creatures is becoming commonplace, but less so in others. It can be difficult to remember what pre-op advice was given to the last owner whose mouse had a lumpectomy, so a written protocol kept in reception will be helpful and saves a lot of frantic thinking.

Post-op

It is important that all these small animals eat as soon as possible after recovery, ideally within 30–60 minutes. Provided that they are kept warm and quiet, have pain relief when necessary and are not dehydrated, the majority will eat within this period.

Dandelions, leaves and flowers, are a good appetite stimulant, especially for rabbits at this time, and practices which regularly treat small furries are recommended to cultivate these plants in the garden or indoors in winter. Forcing plants during late winter and early spring (cover the plant with an upturned flowerpot) encourages the growth of young tender leaves, and regular picking throughout the summer will encourage new growth. Other wild plants and herbs which may be useful for tempting appetites can also be grown in pots, window boxes or in a corner of the garden, where they should be protected from soiling by cats or dogs. The quantities eaten immediately post-op are unlikely to cause digestive upsets, even when these foods are not normally fed.

Animals that have had dental surgery may need puréed food (carrots, dandelions or green vegetables) or vegetarian baby foods which can be syringe fed until they can eat normally.

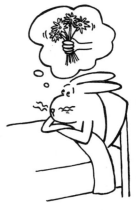

I'm sure I'd feel better if someone brought me some flowers . . . even dandelions would do

And finally, the most important part, without which all your knowledge is useless – owner compliance.

OWNER COMPLIANCE

When recommending any diet for any animal it is not enough to say to the owner, 'Feed this food to your pet'. They must first be convinced that this is the correct and best diet for their pet. Each animal and each owner is an individual, some animals will have more than one owner and the relationship between the animal and each owner may be different, so you have a lot of convincing to do.

Domestic pets are largely dependent on their owners for food. Cats will hunt and dogs will scavenge, but the major part of their diet is supplied and chosen by the owner(s). The Introduction high-lighted the role that food plays in human relationships and in many cases it plays an equally important role in the human–pet relationship. Animals kept as pets are now more important to more people than ever before. They are increasingly regarded as part of the family, 'almost human'. The owner will take as much or more care choosing food for the pet as any other family member, offering that food not just as a cure for hunger but as a measure of their love for it and as a reward for its companionship.

The owner's choice of food is influenced by their perception of the animal's 'likes', the design on the packaging, the most effective advertising blurb and how much they can afford to spend. If the owner does not like the look, smell, feel or cost of a food, the animal doesn't get it. Many of the clinical diets look boring and unappetising; owners expect their pets to interpret being fed these diets as being no longer loved and wanted, and are tempted to add titbits and treats to relieve the 'boredom'.

The argument for variety has already been rehearsed but deserves a second mention here. Humans need to eat a variety of foods to ensure a balanced diet, but a manufactured pet food which contains nutrients and energy appropriate to the species, health status and age of the pet is sufficient and can be fed daily without detriment. From a nutritional point of view I believe this, but as a pet owner I am not so sure. Many owners feel that their pet needs variety and some do in fact appear to do so. Whether this is due to earlier conditioning as a result of the owner's provision of variety or something inherent in the animal, I do not know. Certainly animals have preferences, e.g. dry v. tinned, fish v.

meat, but as a pet owner I am confusing 'like' with 'need'.

'Need' is an essential requirement, 'like' is a preference. Energy and nutrients are essential requirements for life, apple v. pear is a preference. Fortunately most manufacturers now recognize the desire to satisfy both requirement and preference and supply food in two or more varieties.

Owner compliance is particularly important when clinical diets are recommended, as full efficacy cannot be achieved without the cooperation of the owner and the whole family. As we have seen, the temptation is there to add treats or use other products to provide variety when what is really needed is the diet, water and nothing else. There are times when titbits will continue to be fed; in these cases the wisest thing is to limit the damage by suggesting treats which will interfere least with the proposed diet. The art of successful veterinary nursing is to take the theory and scientific fact and blend it into practical reality.

When a pet is ill, particularly when it is seriously ill with perhaps only a short life expectancy, the owner's need to cosset is even greater than normal and the recommendation of special foods must be undertaken with great tact and care. It is probably best at this point to outline the needs of the animal, together with possible ways of supplying these needs, and then let the owner decide on the diet. Slight mismanagement at this stage may shorten life a little but quality of life is more important than ever. A few days enjoying food will be seen in most cases to be better than a few weeks eating boring foods that are poorly accepted. A shorter life but a happier one.

Owner compliance is more likely to be achieved when the client understands the importance of what they are being asked to do, but it needs to be said that not all clients fully understand scientific terminology, so it may be necessary to think laterally and describe the situation in terms that they can understand. On occasions this requires the veterinary nurse to use considerable amounts of imagination, but is worth the effort to ensure the well-being of the pet in question.

Remember:

- the pet is dependent on the owner's choice of food
- the owner's choice depends on *you*.

I know she's on the Hay diet but . . .

Questions

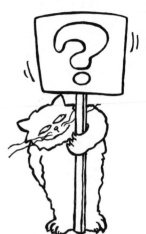

Feeding

1. What are the benefits of caecotrophy?
2. Which nutritionally-related conditions are most commonly seen in rabbits?
3. Name two factors that contribute to obesity in rabbits (and other small furries).
4. Adult rabbits require at least ___ fibre in their diet.
5. Which two rodents kept as pets are strict herbivores?
6. Sunflower seeds, although enjoyed by nearly all rodents, have two major drawbacks and so are best avoided or fed only in small quantities. What are these drawbacks?
7. The digestive system of the chinchilla is designed to cope with a ____ fibre, ____ energy content diet. Adult chinchillas require a fibre level of around ___.
8. How many raisins may be fed to a chinchilla daily?
9. Young chipmunks and pregnant or lactating females require extra protein. How may this be provided?
10. The digestive system of the gerbil is less well designed to cope with _____ amounts of fibre, so this needs to be _____ than in diets for chinchillas, guinea-pigs and rabbits.
11. Gerbils are able to conserve fluids, producing a very concentrated urine and so do not require a water supply. True or false?
12. What does the guinea-pig have in common with humans?
13. Pregnancy toxaemia may occur in guinea-pigs. What additions to the diet help prevent this?
14. Caecal impaction is seen in older guinea-pigs with loss of muscle tone. How can diet help lessen the risk of this condition developing?
15. Hamsters are _____ and when kept as pets are often short of _____ protein. Supplementing the hamster mix with hard-boiled egg, cheese, etc., is particularly important for _____ animals and _____ or _____ females.
16. Diabetes mellitus occurs in _____ hamsters as an inherited condition. It is usually apparent by the age of _____ months. What dietary modifications are necessary for these animals?
17. Young mice and rats and breeding animals require protein levels of around _____. Other adults should be fed a diet with a lower protein content,

as too high levels may lead to ____ problems. Older rats fed too high protein diets are liable to develop _____ _____ _____.

18. Theobromine found in chocolate for human consumption is toxic to _____ and _____ , as well as dogs.

19. Ferrets are carnivores with _____ protein requirements. They have a short gut transit time and require _____ _____ food with a ___ fibre content.

20. Which foods should be offered to maintain the ferret's teeth in good condition?

Hand rearing

1. Why is colostrum important?
2. How many times daily does the rabbit doe normally feed her young?
3. From what age is the hand rearing of chipmunks practical?
4. At what age do ferret kits first take solid food?

Pre- and post-op feeding

1. Like dogs and cats, small furries should be fasted for 12 hours prior to anaesthesia. True or false?
2. Chinchillas, guinea-pigs and rabbits should be fasted for 2–3 hours prior to an operation. Why?
3. Ferrets are able to vomit but need only to be fasted for 4–6 hours as they have a _____ gut transit time.
4. All small animals should eat as soon as possible after recovery, ideally within _____ minutes.
5. Puréed foods may be necessary after _____ surgery.

Bibliography

Anatomy and physiology

Boyd, J.S. (1994). *Color Atlas of Clinical Anatomy of the Dog and Cat*. Mosby.

Clarenburg, R. (1992). *Physiological Chemistry of Domestic Animals*. Mosby.

Engelking, L.R. (2000). *Metabolic and Endocrine Physiology*. Teton NewMedia.

McBride, D.F. (1996). *Learning Veterinary Terminology*. Mosby.

Michell, A.R. (1989). *An Introduction to Veterinary Anatomy and Physiology*. BSAVA.

Nutrition

Benyon, P.H. and Cooper, J.E. (1991). *Manual of Exotic Pets*. BSAVA.

Burger, I. (ed.) (1996). *The Waltham Book of Companion Animal Nutrition*. Pergamon.

Carey, D.P., Norton, S.A. and Bolser, S.M. (1996). *Recent Advances in Canine and Feline Nutritional Research. Proceedings of the 1996 Iams International Nutrition Symposium*. Orange Fraser Press (Ohio).

Case, L.P. (1999). *The Dog, Its Behaviour, Nutrition and Health*. Iowa State University Press/Ames.

Davies, M. (1996). *Canine and Feline Geriatrics*. Blackwell Science.

Flecknell, P. (ed.) (2000). *Manual of Rabbit Medicine and Surgery*. BSAVA.

Gorman, C. (1995). *The Ageing Dog*. Henston.

Hand, M.S., Thatcher, C.D., Remillard, R.L. and Roudebush, P. (2000). *Small Animal Clinical Nutrition*, 4th edn. Mark Morris Associates.

Kelly, N.C. and Wills, J.M. (1996). *Manual of Companion Animal Nutrition and Feeding*. BSAVA.

Laber-Laird, K., Swindle, M.M. and Flecknell, P. (1996). *Handbook of Rabbit and Rodent Medicine*. Pergamon.

Lane, D.R. and Cooper, B. (1999). *Veterinary Nursing*, 2nd edn. Butterworth-Heinemann.

Lewington, J. (2000). *Ferret Husbandry, Medicine and Surgery*. Butterworth-Heinemann.

Lewis, L.D., Morris, M.L. and Hand, M.S. (1987). *Small Animal Clinical Nutrition*, 3rd edn. Mark Morris Associates.

Lloyd, M. (1999). *Ferrets, Health, Husbandry and Diseases*. Blackwell Science.

National Research Council (1985). *Nutrient Requirements of Dogs*. National Academy Press, Washington.

National Research Council (1986). *Nutrient Requirements of Cats*. National Academy Press, Washington.

National Research Council (1995). *Nutrient Requirements of Laboratory Animals*. National Academy Press, Washington.

Okerman, L. (1994). *Diseases of Domestic Rabbits*, 2nd edn. Blackwell Science.

Reinhart, G. and Carey, D.P. (eds) (1998). *Recent Advances in Canine and Feline Nutritional Research*, vol. 2, *Proceedings of the 1998 Iams International Nutrition Symposium*. Orange Fraser Press (Ohio).

Richardson, V.C.G. (1992). *Diseases of Domestic Guinea Pigs*. Blackwell Science.

Richardson, V.C.G. (1997). *Diseases of Small Domestic Rodents*. Blackwell Science.

Richardson, V. (2000). *Rabbits, Health, Husbandry and Diseases*. Blackwell Science.

Simpson, J.W., Anderson, R.S. and Markwell, P. (1993). *Clinical Nutrition of the Dog and Cat*. Blackwell Science.

Strombeck, D.R. (1999). *Home-prepared Dog and Cat Diets*. Iowa State University Press/Ames.

Taylor, D. (1996). *Small Pet Handbook*. HarperCollins.

Williams, D.L. (1998). *Exotic Pets*. Lifelearn.

Wills, J.M. and Simpson, K.W. (1994). *The Waltham Book of Clinical Nutrition of the Dog and Cat*. Pergamon.

Journals

FAB (the quarterly journal of the Feline Advisory Bureau)

Rabbit Healthcare (the Rabbit Charity publication for vets)

Rabbiting On (quarterly magazine of the British House Rabbit Association)

Veterinary International (Friskies Nutrition, Nestec Ltd.)

Veterinary Nursing (journal of the British Veterinary Nursing Association)

Veterinary Practice Nurse

Veterinary Technician (journal of the North American Veterinary Technician Association)

Waltham Focus

FURTHER READING

Anatomy and physiology

Case, L.P. (1999). Digestion and absorption in dogs. In *The Dog, Its Behaviour, Nutrition and Health.* Iowa State University Press/Ames. pp 294–296.

McBride, D.F. (1996). *Learning Veterinary Terminology.* Mosby. pp 207–217.

Maskell, I.E. and Johnson, J.V. (1996). Digestion and absorption. In *The Waltham Book of Companion Animal Nutrition* (I. Burger, ed.). Pergamon. pp 25–44.

Pearson, A.J. (1999). Anatomy and physiology. In *Veterinary Nursing*, 2nd edn (Lane, D.R. and Cooper, B., eds). Butterworth-Heinemann. pp 255–319.

Simpson, J.W., Anderson, R.S. and Markwell, P. (1993). Anatomy and physiology of the digestive tract. In *Clinical Nutrition of the Dog and Cat.* Blackwell Science. pp 1–18.

Components of food

Burger, I. (ed.) (1996). A basic guide to nutrient requirements. In *The Waltham Book of Companion Animal Nutrition.* Pergamon. pp 5–24.

Case, L.P. (1999). Nutrient requirements of the dog. In *The Dog, Its Behaviour, Nutrition and Health.* Iowa State University Press/Ames. pp 277–294.

Gross, K.L., Wedekind, K.J., Cowell, C.S. *et al.* (2000). Nutrients. In *Small Animal Clinical Nutrition*, 4th edn (Hand, M.S., Thatcher, C.D., Remillard, R.L. and Roudebush, P., eds). Mark Morris Associates. pp 21–26, 36–95.

Lewis, L.D., Morris, M.L. and Hand, M.S. (1987). Nutrients. In *Small Animal Clinical Nutrition*, 3rd edn Mark Morris Associates. pp 1-11–1-23.

McCune, S. (1999). Nutrition. In *Veterinary Nursing*, 2nd edn (Lane, D.R. and Cooper, B., eds). Butterworth-Heinemann. pp 171–179.

Simpson, J.W., Anderson, R.S. and Markwell, P. (1993). Nutrients and the requirements of dogs and cats. In *Clinical Nutrition of the Dog and Cat.* Blackwell Science. pp 20–37.

Energy

Gross, K.L., Wedekind, K.J., Cowell, C.S. *et al.* (2000). Nutrients. In *Small Animal Clinical Nutrition*, 4th edn (Hand, M.S., Thatcher, C.D., Remillard, R.L. and Roudebush, P., eds). Mark Morris Associates. pp 25–36.

Lewis, L.D., Morris, M.L. and Hand, M.S. (1987). Nutrients. In *Small Animal Clinical Nutrition,* 3rd edn. Mark Morris Associates. pp 1-3–1-11.

McCune, S. (1999). Nutrition. In *Veterinary Nursing,* 2nd edn (Lane, D.R. and Cooper, B., eds). Butterworth-Heinemann. pp 170–171, 179–180.

Types of food

Burger, I.H. and Thompson, A. (1994). Reading a petfood label. In *The Waltham Book of Clinical Nutrition of the Dog and Cat* (Wills, J.M. and Simpson, K.W., eds). Pergamon. pp 15–23.

Case, L.P. (1999). Diets: evaluation and selection. In *The Dog, Its Behaviour, Nutrition and Health.* Iowa State Univesity Press/Ames. pp 299–305.

Crane, S.W., Griffin, R.W. and Messent, P.R. (2000). Introduction to commercial pet foods. In *Small Animal Clinical Nutrition,* 4th edn (Hand, M.S., Thatcher, C.D., Remillard, R.L. and Roudebush, P., eds). Mark Morris Associates. pp 111–117.

Lewis, L.D., Morris, M.L. and Hand, M.S. (1987). Pet foods. In *Small Animal Clinical Nutrition,* 3rd edn. Mark Morris Associates. pp 2-15–2-16.

McCune, S. (1999). Nutrition. In *Veterinary Nursing,* 2nd edn (Lane, D.R. and Cooper, B., eds). Butterworth-Heinemann. pp 180–182.

Home-made diets

Donoghue, S. and Kronfeld, D.S. (1994). Home-made diets. In *The Waltham Book of Clinical Nutrition of the Dog and Cat* (Wills, J.M. and Simpson, K.W., eds). Pergamon. pp 445–449.

Lewis, L.D., Morris, M.L. and Hand, M.S. (1987). Recipes for homemade dietary foods. In *Small Animal Clinical Nutrition,* 3rd edn. Mark Morris Associates. pp A3-1–A3-3.

Remillard, R.L., Paragon, B., Crane, S.W. *et al.* (2000). Making pet foods at home. In *Small Animal Clinical Nutrition,* 4th edn (Hand, M.S., Thatcher, C.D., Remillard, R.L. and Roudebush, P., eds). Mark Morris Associates. pp 163–178.

Strombeck, D.R. (1999). *Home-prepared Dog and Cat Diets.* Iowa State University Press/Ames.

Feeding dogs and cats

Lewis, D., Morris, M.L. and Hand, M.S. (1987). Enteral feeding. In *Small Animal Clinical Nutrition,* 3rd edn. Mark Morris Associates. pp 5-19–5-34.

McCune, S. (1999). Nutrition. In *Veterinary Nursing,* 2nd edn (Lane, D.R. and Cooper, B., eds). Butterworth-Heinemann. pp 192–193.

Remillard, R.L., Armstrong, P.J. and Davenport, D.J. (2000). Assisted feeding in hospitalised patients. Enteral-assisted feeding. In *Small Animal Clinical Nutrition*, 4th edn (Hand, M.S., Thatcher, C.D., Remillard, R.L. and Roudebush, P., eds). Mark Morris Associates. pp 371–375.

Simpson, J.W., Anderson, R.S. and Markwell, P. (1993). Enteral feeding. In *Clinical Nutrition of the Dog and Cat*. Blackwell Science. pp 101–107.

Lifestage foods

Case, L.P. (1999). Feeding management throughout the life cycle. In *The Dog, Its Behaviour, Nutrition and Health*. Iowa State University Press/Ames. pp 315–324.

Davies, M. (1996). Nutrition in older animals. In *Canine and Feline Geriatrics*. Blackwell Science. pp 112–118.

England, G.C.W. (1999). Obstetric and paediatric nursing of the dog and cat. In *Veterinary Nursing*, 2nd edn (Lane, D.R. and Cooper, B., eds). Butterworth-Heinemann. pp 487–488.

Gorman, C. (1995) Nutrition. In *The Ageing Dog*. Henston. pp 83–96.

Hand, M.S., Thatcher, C.D., Remillard, R.L. and Roudebush, P. (eds) (2000). *Small Animal Clinical Nutrition*, 4th edn. Mark Morris Associates. pp 201–347.

Legrand-Defretin, V. and Munday, H.S. (1996). Feeding dogs and cats for life. In *The Waltham Book of Companion Animal Nutrition* (Burger, I., ed.). Pergamon. pp 57–68.

Lewis, D., Morris, M.L. and Hand, M.S. (1987). Dogs – feeding and care. Cats – feeding and care. In *Small Animal Clinical Nutrition*, 3rd edn. Mark Morris Associates. pp 3-2–3-31; 4-1–4-12.

McCune, S. (1999). Nutrition. In *Veterinary Nursing*, 2nd edn (Lane, D.R. and Cooper, B., eds). Butterworth-Heinemann. pp 183–190.

McLaughlin, S. (1998). Feeding for gestation and lactation in the bitch. *Veterinary Nursing*, **13**, 135–137.

Mullane, P.A. (1998). Practical neonatal care: tube feeding. *Veterinary Technician*, **19**, 532–534.

Simpson, J.W., Anderson, R.S. and Markwell, P. (1993). Nutrition and old age. In *Clinical Nutrition of the Dog and Cat*. Blackwell Science. pp 115–127.

The gut as an ecosystem

Buddington, R.K. and Sunvold, G.D. (1998). Fermentable fibre and the gastrointestinal tract ecosystem. In *Recent Advances in Canine and Feline Nutritional Research*, Vol. 2, *Proceedings of the 1998 Iams Nutrition Symposium* (Reinhart, G. and Carey, D.P., eds). Orange Fraser Press (Ohio).

Schoenherr, W.D., Roudebush, P. and Swecker, W.S. (2000). Use of fatty acids in inflammatory disease. In *Small Animal Clinical Nutrition*, 4th edn (Hand, M.S., Thatcher, C.D., Remillard, R.L. and Roudebush, P., eds). Mark Morris Associates. pp 907–911.

Clinical nutrition

Bucher, L. (1998). Meeting the dietary needs of pets with cancer. *Veterinary Practice Nurse*, **10**, 11–12.

Case, L.P. (1999). Common nutrition problems in dogs. In *The Dog, Its Behaviour, Nutrition and Health*. Iowa State University Press/Ames. pp 331–346.

Hand, M.S., Thatcher, C.D., Remillard, R.L. and Roudebush, P. (eds) (2000). In *Small Animal Clinical Nutrition*, 4th edn. Mark Morris Associates. pp 351–939.

Lewis, D., Morris, M.L. and Hand, M.S. (1987). Chapters 5 to 12. In *Small Animal Clinical Nutrition*, 3rd edn. Mark Morris Associates.

McCune, S. (1999). Nutrition. In *Veterinary Nursing*, 2nd edn (Lane, D.R. and Cooper, B., eds). Butterworth-Heinemann. pp 194–201.

Simpson, J.W., Anderson, R.S. and Markwell, P. (1993). Nutritional diseases. Dietary management of clinical diseases. In *Clinical Nutrition of the Dog and Cat*. Blackwell Science. pp 39–53; 56–91.

Sturgess, K. (1999). Chronic renal failure in cats, what role for nutrition? *FAB*, **37**, 22–25.

Wills, J.M. and Simpson, K.W. (1994). Part 1 Principles of clinical nutrition, Part 2 Clinical nutrition in practice. In *The Waltham Book of Clinical Nutrition of the Dog and Cat*. Pergamon.

Small furries

Barwick, R. (2000). Rabbit nutrition. *Veterinary Nursing*, **15**, 94–100.

Carpenter, J.W. and Kolmstetter, C.M. (2000). Feeding small exotic pets. In *Small Animal Clinical Nutrition*, 4th edn (Hand, M.S., Thatcher, C.D., Remillard, R.L. and Roudebush, P., eds). Mark Morris Associates. pp 943–959.

Cooper, J.E. and Dutton, C.J. (1999). Exotic pets and wildlife. In *Veterinary Nursing*, 2nd edn (Lane, D.R. and Cooper, B., eds). Butterworth-Heinemann. pp 216–219; 224–229.

Harcourt-Brown, F. (1998). Feeding pet rabbits. *Veterinary Practice Nurse*, **10**, 4–7.

Lloyd, M. (1999). Nutrition. Nutritional diseases. In *Ferrets, Health, Husbandry and Diseases*. Blackwell Science. pp 18–20; 116–119.

Lewington, J. (2000). *Ferret Husbandry, Medicine and Surgery*. Butterworth-Heinemann.

McCune, S. (1999). Nutrition. In *Veterinary Nursing*, 2nd edn. (Lane, D.R. and Cooper, B., eds). Butterworth-Heinemann. pp 201–203.

Meredith, A. (2000). Anatomy and biology, diet. In *Manual of Rabbit Medicine and Surgery* (Flecknell, P., ed). BSAVA. pp 16–18, 21.

Richardson, V.C.G. (1992). The digestive system. Nutrition. In *Diseases of Domestic Guinea Pigs*. Blackwell Science. pp 49–60; 86–96.

Richardson, V.C.G. (1997). Chinchillas, nutrition. The digestive system. Chipmunks, nutrition. The digestive system. Gerbils, nutrition. The digestive system. Hamsters, nutrition. The digestive system. Mice, nutrition. The digestive system. Rats, nutrition. The digestive system. In *Diseases of Small Domestic Rodents*. Blackwell Science. pp 4–7; 26–33; 56–57; 62–63; 77–78; 88–92; 112–114; 125–132; 154–156; 165–167; 190–192; 202–205.

Richardson, V. (2000). Nutrition. The digestive system. In *Rabbits, Health, Husbandry and Diseases*. Blackwell Science. pp 7–18; 81–107.

Taylor, D. (1996). Food for the small pet. In *Small Pet Handbook*. HarperCollins. pp 68–80.

Answers

COMPONENTS OF FOOD

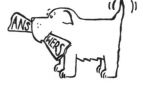

1. 10%.
2. The oxidation of carbohydrate, fat and protein.
3. False. Cell repair and replacement is a continuous process and needs a continuous supply of the essential amino acids.
4. False. Taurine, an essential amino acid for the cat, is only found in animal tissue.
5. A protein catalyst involved in many metabolic reactions.
6. Linoleic, linolenic and arachidonic acids.
7. Short chains of monosaccharides which can be hydrolysed to simple sugars but often act as fibre.
8. Biotin.
9. Hundred (10 g/kg diet). Million (1 mg/kg diet).
10. Antioxidants neutralize free radicals and help prevent damage to tissues.

ENERGY

1. Resting.
2. Faecal. Digestible
3. Metabolizable.
4. Puppies and kittens have high energy requirements but have very limited stomach capacity.
5. Acceptability, energy needs and palatability.

TYPES OF FOOD

1. Lightly. Salt. Variety. Adequate.
2. Complete. Complementary. Complete diets may be fed alone.

3. Syrup.
4. True. The animal will drink more to compensate for the lower water content of dry food.
5. Dry weight. Energy content.

FEEDING DOGS AND CATS

1. False. Overweight pups will be overweight adults.
2. Feeding on demand.
3. True.
4. Enteral.
5. Artificial feeding is necessary when the animal cannot be persuaded to eat voluntarily as without food the animal will become nutritionally compromised.
6. The provision of adequate nutrients by intravenous catheter.

LIFESTAGE FOODS

1. Between 1:1 and 1.5:1.
2. True.
3. True.
4. False. Pregnant and lactating bitches will require energy-dense food in the last weeks of pregnancy and the first 3–4 weeks of lactation. Toy dogs, nervous dogs and finicky eaters may also benefit from energy-dense foods. A watch should always be kept on weight and body condition.
5. It is nutritionally balanced for that species. Maternal antibodies are passed to the neonate together with other proteins which encourage correct development of the immature gut. It provides hormones, growth factors and enzymes which promote correct growth and development of the animal.
6. Three to four.
7. False. Many animals lose the ability to digest milk efficiently after weaning. Ingestion of milk may then lead to digestive upsets.
8. Exercise. Skeletal.

THE GUT AS AN ECOSYSTEM

1. Bacteria, Fungi, Protozoa, Yeasts.
2. Bifidobacteria, Eubacteria, Lactobacilli.
3. The edging out of one species by another.

4. Substances which alter the gut flora in favour of beneficial microorganisms.
5. Compounds derived from polyunsaturated fatty acids which act as a type of hormone and regulate normal physiology.

CLINICAL NUTRITION

Obesity

1. 20%. Females. Males.
2. A decreased. Maintaining.
3. A decrease. An increase.

Starvation

1. True. Although skeletal muscle is lost in preference to the muscle of internal organs, loss of protein from skeletal muscle is almost always accompanied by a degree of internal protein loss.
2. It should be checked for hydration status and fluid levels restored if necessary.
3. Protein-energy malnutrition. An accelerated form of starvation.
4. True. Many of the body tissues are able to use fat and protein for energy, tumour cells cannot do this.

Skeletal disease

1. False. These conditions usually occur in young, growing animals but may also be seen in older animals.
2. Oxalate and phytate are constituents of plants which bind with calcium and prevent its absorption by the body.
3. Phosphorus. Calcium. Rickets. Osteomalacia.
4. Glucosamine, Chondroitin.

Neuromuscular disease

1. True.
2. Protein. Muscle mass.
3. Correct deficiencies. Restore correct function.

Disorders of the integument

1. True. Similar symptoms can occur for a variety of reasons.
2. 30. Skin. Hair. Relative. Lactation. Low.
3. A minimum of 6 weeks.
4. Over-supplementation should be avoided to avoid excesses which can be as damaging as deficiencies and to prevent further upsets in nutrient balance.
5. When dietary intolerance or hypersensitivity is suspected in either skin or intestinal conditions.

Cardiovascular disease

1. Taurine. True.
2. Drug.
3. Calorie density.

Digestive system

1. Reguritation. Vomiting.
2. Motility, secretion and digestion.
3. True. Two examples are travel sickness and uraemia arising as a result of disease elsewhere in the body.
4. Food. Inflammation. Colitis. Colon.
5. Absorption of nutrients takes place mainly in the small intestine and interference with this uptake can have serious consequences for the animal.
6. Faecal volume. Water content.
7. Endocrine. Exocrine. Exocrine. Sodium bicarbonate. Enzymes.
8. Exocrine pancreatic insufficiency. Steatorrhoea.
9. If these enzymes were secreted in an active form they would digest the pancreas itself. When protective mechanisms break down, the enzymes can become active in the pancreas giving rise to pancreatitis.
10. Portosystemic shunt.
11. Bedlington terriers.
12. False. There are three types of jaundice, of which only hepatic jaundice is due to primary liver disease. Pre- and post-hepatic types of jaundice are due to other factors.

Reproductive system

1. True.
2. Bitches. Small. Peak lactation.

Urinary system

1. False. These symptoms can occur in other diseases and problems. They usually require further investigation when reported by the owner.
2. Infection, Nephrotoxins, Shock, Dehydration, Trauma, Obstruction.
3. Chronic renal failure.
4. Renal secondary hyperparathyroidism.
5. Pain. Discomfort. Frequently. Smaller. Blood.
6. False. Calcium oxalate and silicate uroliths require surgical removal.

Endocrine system

1. Insulin is the major hormone involved in lowering blood glucose levels. It also has a role to play in the metabolism of fats and protein.
2. Slows. Fluctuations.
3. True.
4. Increased energy density to restore lost weight. Most affected cats are older animals so protein and fat levels should be appropriate for geriatric cats. Dietary requirements for other, concurrent illness should be considered.

SMALL FURRIES

Feeding

1. The animal is able to obtain more nutrients from the food and is able to economize on water intake.
2. Dental problems and obesity.
3. Overfeeding of concentrate rations and lack of exercise.
4. 20%.
5. Chinchillas and guinea-pigs.
6. Sunflower seeds are high in fat and low in calcium.
7. High. Low. 30%.
8. No more than two.
9. Hard-boiled egg, cheese, milk powder, crickets or mealworms.
10. Large. Lower.
11. False. Although they drink very little, clean, fresh water should always be available, particularly when no fresh food is offered.

12. Both guinea-pigs and humans are unable to synthesize vitamin C. This must be provided in the diet on a daily basis.
13. A small amount of glucose added to the drinking water and calcium supplementation in the last week of pregnancy and first week of lactation.
14. Adequate levels of fibre (around 15%) should be provided and care taken not to overfeed.
15. Omnivorous. Animal. Young. Pregnant. Lactating.
16. Chinese. Three. Sweet foods, fruits and young leaves should not be fed. A slight increase in fibre levels is often beneficial.
17. 24%. Skin. Chronic renal failure.
18. Rats. Ferrets.
19. High. Highly digestible. Low.
20. Tough meat, dry food or hard biscuits will help maintain dental health.

Hand rearing

1. Colostrum contains antibodies which provide passive immunity and other hormones, growth factors, etc., which greatly increase the neonates' chances of survival. These factors are not present in milk substitutes.
2. Once or sometimes twice daily.
3. From the age of one week.
4. Between 14 and 21 days.

Pre- and post-op feeding

1. False. These animals have only small reserves of protein and energy and have a high metabolic rate. Fasting induces a catabolic state and is unnecessary as most do not vomit.
2. After a large meal a full stomach may impinge on the thoracic cavity, reducing lung capacity and increasing anaesthetic hazards. Allowing a short period of fasting ensures that the stomach is not too enlarged.
3. Rapid.
4. 30–60.
5. Dental.

Index